THE HEART OF HOSPICE

Dedication

This book is lovingly dedicated to my dearest friend, **Donalda McGeachy**, and to all her caregivers.

> *Spiritual care lies at the heart of hospice. It says we are here. We will be with you in your living and your dying. We will free you from pain and give you the freedom to find your own meaning in your own life – your way. We will comfort you and those you love – not always with words, often with a touch or a glance. We will bring you hope – not for tomorrow but for this day. We will not leave you. We will watch with you. We will be there.*

Dorothy Ley

Dedicated to the memory of Dorothy Ley and Iris Man: two women of extraordinary courage, compassion and faith. Their lessons will live on through their words, their example and our memories.

Harry van Bommel

THE HEART OF HOSPICE

Dorothy C.H. Ley
with Harry van Bommel

NC Press Limited
Toronto 1994

To contact Harry van Bommel for speaking engagements, write or call:
PSD Consultants
11 Miniot Circle
Scarborough, Ontario, Canada
M1K 2K1
(416) 264-4665

Canadian Cataloguing in Publication Data

Main Entry under title:
The Heart of Hospice

(FAMILYbooks)
Includes bibliographical references and index.
ISBN 155021-087-4

1. Hospice care - Canada. 2. Hospice care.
I. van Bommel, Harry. II Title. III Series.

R726.8.L48 1993 362.1'75 C93-09527-X

We would like to thank the Ontario Arts Council, the Ontario Publishing Centre, the Ontario Ministry of Culture, Tourism and Recreation, the Canada Council and the Government of Canada, Department of Communications for their assistance in the production of this book.

New Canada Publications, a division of NC Press Limited, Box 452, Station A, Toronto, Ontario, Canada, M5W 1H8.

Printed and bound in Canada

Contents

Acknowledgements

by Harry van Bommel

Dorothy would have wanted the following people thanked for taking such good care of her both at home and in the hospital (in alphabetical order): **Dr. Harold Ames**, **Betty Ballard**, **Doreen Berry**, **Dorothy Bircher**, **Norma** and **Bill Brown**, **Dr. Jose Chan**, **Ron Coovadia**, **Charlotte Empringham**, **Susie Galiegue**, **Dr. Gillian Gilchrist**, **Ann Link**, **Dr. Pat Marchuk**, **Barbara** and **John McGeachy**, **Geoffrey** and **Mary Parke-Taylor**, **Marlene Siomra**, the entire palliative care team and the staff on the main floor at Oshawa General Hospital, and the St. Elizabeth Visiting Nurses Association who attended Dorothy at home.

I would like to add my personal thanks to many of the people listed above who spent time with me telling me stories filled with love, laughter and insight about their friend Dorothy Ley. Their efforts form a large part of the biographical sketch that appears in this book. I would like to add thanks to **Norma Clarke**, **Don Foster**, **Shirley Herron**, **Marilyn Lundy** and **Meade Wright** for their invaluable contributions.

Caroline Walker, publisher of NC Press Limited was always excited about this book's possibilities and patient throughout the long delays in getting the book ready for production. Caroline, through her quiet, ongoing support of Canadian hospice care continues to provide us with books that deal with this, and other, important social issues. I am grateful to her for her foresight.

Kathy Bowden, **Norman Endicott**, **Shirley Herron** and **Janet Walker** reviewed a draft of this book and I am most indebted to them for their editorial advice and interest in this project. A special thank you to **Andrew Martindale** of NC Press Limited for the excellent typesetting and actual production of this book. His unique perspective has added to the book's overall quality. **Waneta Storms** has been instrumental in making the Canadian public aware of Dr. Ley's work.

I would like to thank the *Journal of Palliative Care* for permission to reproduce their logo on our back cover and throughout this text. This logo was designed during the time that Dorothy Ley was head of the Palliative Care Foundation and she was instrumental in its development. The symbol is a twentieth century printer's linotype ornament. It was chosen as a logo because it contains the elements that effectively communicate the objectives of the Journal. The ornament consists mainly of two parts united to form one harmonious unit. The inner part of the ornament suggests the waves of the sea (which has commonly symbolized life itself) while the other area suggests the appearance of a gentle, protective circle (similar to the function of palliative care). The whole suggests the restorative qualities associated with the sea uplifting the human spirit. This connotes the same idea that good palliative care can maintain the dignity and self- respect of the patient and the family.

We would also like to acknowledge that portions of this book are taken from a chapter by Dr. Ley that first appeared as: "Spiritual Care in Hospice" in *Death and Spirituality* edited by Kenneth J. Koka with John D. Morgan. (1992). Amityville, NY: Baywood Publishing Company, Inc.

We further acknowledge permission to reproduce, in the Appendix to this book, the Assumptions and Principles of Spiritual Care; A Statement of Assumptions and Principles Concerning Education About Death, Dying and Bereavement; and A Statement of Assumptions and Principles Concerning Education About Death, Dying and Bereavement for Professionals in Health Care and Human Services, produced, with Dr. Ley's participation, by The International Work Group on Death, Dying and Bereavement. Further information on their work is available at: the International Work Group Secretariat, King's College, 266 Epworth Avenue, London, Ontario, Canada N6A 2M3 (Tel: 519-432-7946).

Special thanks to the Ontario Palliative Care Association for allowing us to reproduce tributes to Dr. Ley published in their *Spring 1994 Special Patron's Issue* (Volume IV, No 1.). These tributes appear with other ones at the beginning of this book. Dr. Ley was the patron of this association and touched the lives of many of its members.

Special thanks also to **The Right Reverend Terrance Finlay**, **Reverend Douglas Graydon**, **Dr. Elizabeth Latimer**, **Dr. Larry Librach**, and **The Right Reverend Geoffrey Parke-Taylor** for permission to quote from their tributes to Dr. Ley at her funeral and memorial services. These tributes appear at the end of the book.

Marlene Siomra, a good friend of Dorothy Ley, painted the portrait of Dr. Ley that appears on the front cover. Dr. Ley was most pleased to see the portrait and a draft sample of the cover before her death.

Half the royalties of *The Heart of Hospice* will be donated to The Dorothy Ley Hospice in Etobicoke, Ontario.

Janet Klees has provided physical, emotional, spiritual and editorial support throughout this project. Like the two women named in my dedication of this book, Janet represents the hospice care philosophy of compassionate support and care on a daily basis to all people she encounters. Her support has made this book possible in more ways than I can describe. Thank you Janet.

Preface

by Harry van Bommel

When Dorothy Ley and I agreed to write this book I predicted, "This is going to be fun." Her reply: "It better be or it isn't worth doing," and then she laughed. We were seated in her hospital room several days after she had received another round of chemotherapy for her cancer. Her mood was uplifted yet peaceful. There were things she wanted to get done but there was also time to just chit chat about family, politics and the summer of '93.

In 1992 I first asked Dorothy to write a book about her views on palliative care. I knew of no one else in Canada who had her unique qualifications to write such a book. There are many leaders in the field of palliative care but only one, that I knew of, who had the perspectives of being a doctor (haematologist, oncologist and palliative care pioneer), a family member who cared for loved ones at home, and a patient with a diagnosis of a terminal illness. Dorothy Ley had all these experiences and, therefore, a unique perspective to pass on to other patients, family members and palliative care-givers.

Originally the content of the entire book was to be Dorothy's. Because of her illness, she was unable to complete a draft of the book. Therefore, on her request, I have completed it in what I hope would be the spirit of her own writing. This book is not exactly what Dorothy and I envisioned when we began but it does serve as her advice to us on what she felt was most important for successful palliative care to exist and flourish in Canada. The book is also a tribute to her as a pioneer in the field of Canadian and international palliative care. In taking care of others we must not forget to take care of each other and remember the leaders of our philosophy of palliative care.

The biographical sketch of Dorothy Ley in this book is important because I believe that people must get to know the person behind the professional, even if only briefly. This is not only true of Dorothy, but of all the leaders in the field of palliative care. We must respect the professionals, volunteers, patients and family members who have been instrumental in developing palliative care in Canada. At the same time, however, we must recognize them as people who need the same kinds of emotional, spiritual and informational supports that all people involved in caring for people who are ill need. Putting them on a pedestal to admire or criticize is unfair to them and unfair to us. Unfair to us because putting people on pedestals permits us to avoid the responsibilities of accomplishing the same tasks with the same compassion and dedication. When we are all on level ground we can work together. This benefits us all individually and benefits society and palliative care as a whole.

As a writer I have promised myself not to work on books with other people because the experience is usually one filled with frustration, ego battles and last minute compromises to the integrity of the text. None of that has occurred with this book. I thoroughly enjoyed working with Dorothy to create a useful educational tool, primarily for use by palliative care providers, but also for everyone interested in palliative care. I also enjoyed our walks around her beautiful home on the shores of Ontario's Lake Simcoe, our chats in her wood panelled office-library about each other's families, our discussions about past successes and our hopes for the future. Her insights are practical, direct, humorous, colourful and inspirational. Her experiences lend a practicality and a credibility to this work that is hard to find elsewhere. Best of all, we can learn from someone who actually practiced what she taught. She was a very human role model to physicians, other health care providers, family members and now to patients. I am grateful for this experience.

Her book is divided into three parts. The first part includes the Introduction and the two chapters on the pillars of care and Dr. Ley's personal comments to people within palliative care. Her words are a compilation of various speeches and articles that she wrote over the years about the importance of providing physical, emotional, spiritual, and informational supports to people with a life-threatening or terminal illness and their families. **They are her words** supplemented by information collected during our conversations together. Part II describes some hospice care success stories including the excellent hospice care that Dr. Ley received in her last months of life. Part III is a collection of information that readers may find helpful in understanding both Dorothy Ley and her message.

Her book is called *The Heart of Hospice* which she saw as the often forgotten spiritual element to palliative care. In a real sense, her belief in, and promotion of, palliative care and her experiences as a doctor, family member and patient put her at the heart of hospice as well – a well deserved place in the history of this young movement in Canada.

NOTE: One of Dorothy's friends found an old, 3.5 x 5 inch notebook that Dorothy must have used decades ago to collect favourite quotes. She entitled her notebook, "Happiness Must Be Earned." There were one hundred quotations in all by many different authors touching on subjects of love, death and dying, character, spirituality, philosophy, loneliness, memories and nature. There were several writers quoted more than once including Joyce Kilmer, Edna St. Vincent Millay, L. M. Bowman, Rudyard Kipling, Robert Frost, Henry Wadsworth Longfellow and Sara Teasdale. I have taken a selection of these quotes and used them as the beginning of some chapters.

Tributes

When Dorothy Ley died on January 31, 1994 there was an outpouring of personal and professional tributes to her. The following is a selection of those tributes. At the end of this book are tributes made to her at her funeral and memorial services in Beaverton and Toronto.

Dorothy Ley demonstrated unfailing compassion and concern for everyone with whom she came in contact in her professional and personal life. A brilliant physician and always keenly aware of her own humanity and that of her patients and coworkers. She had a unique ability to make her patients feel very special to her. Because of this she was very special to each of them.

Norma Clark
Daughter of a Patient

I have known Dorothy over the years in many capacities – professionally, as a pioneer in palliative care; in community work in Durham Region; as a valued friend, generous in her caring and support; and finally as a patient. Much has been said and written about her many accomplishments and the honours which accrued to her in her church and professional life, but it is as a person that I will remember her. Just as hospital, hospice and hospitality, coming from one Latin root, epitomized Dorothy's life and work, so do the words grace, gracefulness and graciousness exemplify her character. When I think of Dorothy, I also think of the words integrity and dignity. Those of us who were privilege to travel the last mile with her and who witnessed her courage as she became less and less able to perform the tasks of daily living, were constantly amazed by her acceptance of the indignity and helplessness. Life was very precious to her – a gift – to be lived to the fullest, but she was one of the fortunate ones who was able to say to me, "I have done everything I wanted to do." – not resignation, but an affirmation of life. It was doubtful at one time if she would be able to accomplish her wish to die at home, but that was made possible by dedicated family, friends and nurses. She died with grace and dignity in her own home with those she loved and who loved her. We are honoured to have known her. Go with God Dorothy.

Dr. Gillian Gilchrist
Medical Director
Palliative Care Team
Oshawa General Hospital

My first association with Dorothy Ley was as a young nurse being "cared for" by Dr. Ley. I was her patient and her care went beyond the usual medical requirements. It was characterized by compassion and by making herself available in her home on weekends or on vacation – whenever care was required. She practised the principles of palliative care long before the words were known. Dorothy later became a mentor, a model and a friend.

Shirley Herron, B.Sc.N.

Dorothy is a beautifully groomed, crisp, articulate, poised, straightforward woman who used to specialize in haematology and oncology. She has seen some two thousand people die, from which experience she has developed a passion for palliative care. She believes that death should be allowed more dignity and humanity than hospital procedures usually permit… "You realize we're talking about a middle-class phenomenon. Palliative care goes to people who have relatives and friends who care about them, but bag ladies die, too. All the dispossessed and lonely need palliative care, and where are they going to get it?"

June Callwood
extract from *Twelve Weeks in Spring* (1986)

I met Dr. Dorothy Ley when the Palliative Care Foundation was established. She was a woman of remarkable energy, commitment and vision. She understood the world of academic medicine, and the need for innovative educational programs, a professional journal and bibliographic resources to develop the knowledge base of a fledging field. She understood the needs of small floundering programs; and, the need for networking and technical support. Most of all, she understood the plight of individual people, patients and family members who needed an advocate. Palliative care in Canada owes much to her charismatic, sound pioneer leadership. She will be sorely missed.

Ina Cummings M.D., C.C.F.P.
Vice-President, Canadian Palliative Care Association
Director, Palliative Care Program
Camp Hill Hospital, Halifax

Dr. Dorothy Ley had a very lengthy struggle with cancer and experienced first hand the troubles, trials and frustrations of a terminal illness. During the final months of her life she was working on a book to share with us some of her experiences and some of the lessons learned on her journey. Her hope was, through her book, to teach more about palliative/hospice care from the recipient's perspective. She has a message for all of us. Dorothy was a remarkable lady who gave unselfishly of her time and her many talents. . . Dorothy loved the people of her community. This was very evident at her funeral. The little church was filled to overflowing and the people who were there to pay their respects came from every walk of life – a tribute to a friend whose life touched so many in her ministries to people, both through medicine and through the church. Ever the caregiver, Dorothy continued to meet people's needs by allowing her many friends to say goodbye in the privacy of their own community.

Shari Douglas
President
Ontario Palliative Care Association

Dr. Dorothy Ley made a very great contribution to palliative care in Canada. She headed the team whose survey of Canadian and international developments led to the establishment of the Palliative Care Foundation (now replaced by the CPCA). As Executive Director of the

Foundation she helped uncounted groups to organize palliative care and hospice services all across this country. I consider her one of the founding mothers of Hospice, along with Cecily Saunders and Elizabeth Kubler-Ross.

Dr. Paul Hentileff
President
Canadian Palliative Care Association (CPCA)

Dorothy reached out to those of us who knew her in very special ways – each way unique to the individual needs we had. Her gift to me was one of friendship. I also value what she shared with me in knowledge and hopefulness of achieving the best of care for palliative care patients and their families. Her shoes will be hard to fill.

Marilyn Lundy, R.N., P.H.N.

In palliative care I have had the opportunity to meet people who leave a lasting impression on my life just by being themselves. Dr. Dorothy Ley was such a person. We first met in the early 70s and she became my model and mentor in palliative care. Whenever I discussed my plans and ideas she always reminded me, "Reena, remember whom you are doing this for. Keep the patient and family the centre of your focus." During her illness we became closer and talked on the phone often. I was inspired by her courage and zest for life. She was a woman of Faith and often talked about spirituality as the heart of palliative/hospice care. She never wavered in her commitment to and interest in palliative care. Her loss to the movement is great. Her loss to me is painful. But for palliative care and for me, Dorothy has left a rich legacy of commitment to the dream and courage in times of adversity, Faith in a powerful God and honesty to ourselves.

Ms. Reena McDermott
Past President
Ontario Palliative Care Association

With the death of Dorothy Ley at her home in Beaverton, Ontario on Monday, January 31, 1994, Canadian Palliative Care has lost a pioneer and one of its most effective protagonists. Dorothy was a richly talented person accustomed to breaking new ground in her multiple careers. As a haematologist/oncologist on the academic staff of the University of Toronto she became the first woman to head a clinical department at the Western Hospital. Subsequent initiatives found her establishing a chain of medical testing laboratories, founding the Canadian Palliative Care Foundation, and lending her energies to a variety of organizations and agencies established to improve the lot of the dying and their families. I didn't always agree with Dorothy. In fact, we frequently found ourselves taking opposite position on questions of mutual concern. In agreement, one found her to be a staunch ally; in disagreement, a most effective debater from whom one stood to learn a great deal. Dorothy touched and enriched the lives of thousands through her tireless industry, her capacity to give, her ready warmth and her spirited dynamism. Thank you, Dorothy, for your many gifts to us. We have lost a champion. We have lost a respected colleague. We have lost a friend.

Dr. Balfour M. Mount
Director of Palliative Care Medicine
McGill University, Montreal

Dorothy Ley will be remembered for her honesty and enduring courage. She was a women with deep commitment to her Christian beliefs and values which were clearly evident at meetings. We will miss Dorothy as an advocate, colleague and friend in the pursuit of palliative care in Canada.

Nora M. O'Donnell
Executive Director
Ottawa-Carleton Regional Palliative Care Association

I am entering my tenth year as editor of the Journal of Palliative Care. *Both the Journal and my editorship would never have happened without Dr. Ley. When she first asked me to work with her and others at the Canadian Palliative Care Foundation to start the Journal, I declined, too busy was I. But Dorothy, like some lovable Welsh terriers I know, would not let go. She convinced me that I should commit myself to palliative care as best I could. That would be as editor of a journal, she thought. Dorothy pointed to a road at a fork in the woods. I am deeply happy that I took that road. So, indeed, how could I ever forget Dr. Ley, as memorable as she will always be for all the wonderful things she had done. When I think of her I recall the workmen's chant in one of T.S. Elliot's poems: "In the vacant place We will build with new bricks.... Where the bricks are fallen We will build with new stone.... Where the word is unspoken We will build with new speech." Dorothy, master manager, rallied us to build with new speech.*

Dr. David Roy
Editor-in-Chief
Journal of Palliative Care

A person of several careers and multiple accomplishments, Dr. Dorothy Ley came to Palliative Care in 1981 offering a rich blend of clinical knowledge, political skills, business acumen and personal energy. Dorothy brought us "guts!" – she was not afraid to tackle anyone or anything. She was fiercely loyal to the church, to her friends and to palliative care. Through her many projects and associations, she advocated for the care of the elderly and the dying and gave Ontario Palliative care an international profile. I join her many friends and colleagues in this tribute to her courage and achievements.

Dr. John F. Scott
Director, Ottawa Regional Palliative Care Unit
Head, Division of Palliative Medicine
University of Ottawa

Dorothy Ley was a sensitive, empathetic lady. She had a vision to improve care of the dying. She was a pioneer, and her dream was to ensure that palliative care principles were practised. Her insight into care of the aged paved a pathway in that area as well. Personal choice was paramount to Dorothy Ley's practice and she encouraged the movement away from a medically dominated model of care. To have known Dorothy was indeed a blessing.

Connie Smith
Nurse Manager/PC Coordinator
Kincardine and District General Hospital

I have had the privilege of knowing Dr. Dorothy Ley for more than ten years in connection with the palliative care movement in Canada, in which she has been both a pioneer and charismatic leader. Her interest in palliative care grew out of her chosen medical speciality Haematology-Oncology. Because of her deep concern for her patients she was aware that many of them were going to die and thus the best that modern medicine had to offer was not enough. From her own spiritual journey she felt driven to lead the growing palliative care movement to a less medically oriented model; while accepting good control of physical symptoms as important, a central place must be left for the spiritual and psycho-social care of the individual. This was clearly demonstrated in her involvement in the development of the new [Ontario] Provincial Palliative Care Initiatives. While representing the Metro Toronto Health Council and being very ill herself, she was a strong voice for the involvement of spiritual care providers and volunteers in pain and symptom management teams. She also felt strongly that education for family physicians and other health care providers should be integrated at the local level. In conclusion, Dorothy will be greatly missed for her wise and impassioned counsel in these changing times, in a rapidly evolving discipline.

Dr. John Swift
Medical Director, Palliative Care
Parkwood Hospital, London Ontario

Dorothy came into my life so very quickly and with such a force of gentleness, serenity, firmness and wisdom. She left too quickly yet stays with me as few have ever done or will. I had the privilege to work with Dorothy on the [Ontario] Provincial Steering Committee for Palliative Care Initiatives. She touched, charged, energized, enriched and strengthened each of us and all of us together. We unanimously agreed that Dorothy should write the Forward to our report. She did. In early 1993, Dorothy told me that her great hope was that she would complete her work in our report. In characteristic fashion, Dorothy had the last word in her Forward to the Report: "The success or failure of these initiatives will depend on the willingness of professionals, volunteers, the public and patients and their families to understand, to cooperate and to support the goals of palliative care." Dorothy continues to challenge and urge us to do those things she did so very well – understand, cooperate and support. Thank you, Dorothy; I miss you.

Gail Ure
Manager, Long Term Care
London, Ontario Office

Biographical Sketch

of Dorothy Corinne Hobbs Ley, M.D., F.R.C.P.(C)., F.A.C.P.

by Harry van Bommel

Out of the Wilderness

I am a renegade, laughing at rules and laws
And my whims are my king and my royal family.

I am an adventurer delving in joy and sorrow
And love and friendship and the white quarries of truth.

I am a plunderer, taking all that the sages have left me
And adding thereto, that the children to come may have peace.

I am a highwayman, stealing the gold of the dawn
And the star-heavy, blue-purple robe of the night.

I hold up the wind for its fragrance and wrestle the sea.
With my brown, naked arms, for the tang of its salt.

I am a pirate, a gay, laughing, profligate pirate
Sailing the seas of delight, where my loot
Is diamonds of sunlight, and the cold pearls of the moon.

Wilson MacDonald

When you meet a person for the first time you usually meet only part of that person: the part that is public and represents the career person. The other part is often hidden from view and is the adult version of the child that was. A curriculum vitae presents the public person's history and accomplishments. At the end of this book is Dorothy's formal history of professional qualifications, volunteer work, awards and a list of her published works.

This chapter, however, looks at the person that grew out of the child born at Toronto General Hospital on April 4, 1924. Her mother Inez Corinne Dunlop (Ley) and her father Charles Thomas Hobbs Ley were both proud of the accomplishments of the little baby that came to them that spring, five short years after World War I. Dorothy grew up in Toronto and her experiences are shaped by that city. During her youth, Toronto was still in its infancy as a modern metropolis. Up to the Second World War, Toronto was primarily populated with White Anglo-Saxon Protestants and that is the environment in which Dorothy grew up. Through her lifetime she had seen it shift from a WASP city to what the United Nations has called the most multi-cultural city in the world. Toronto has people from over 100 countries living with 3,500,000 other people. Catholicism is now the predominate religion and few people take for granted that the leadership within the city will remain in the "old boy," white, middle-to-upper classes beyond the next decade.

Dorothy's childhood was fairly typical of the time. She missed out on some of the normal aspects of childhood because she was so good academically that most of her time was spent reading and learning. In 1940 Dorothy went to the University of Toronto to study literature. Originally she had wanted to study archaeology but the war in Europe and Africa was destroying many of the major archaeological sites in the world. Adapting to the situation, she wanted to be a writer and study the great works of authors from around the world. Early in her studies at Victoria College, however, she discovered that she could complete her week's assignments in one day and soon became bored.

Dorothy was examining several other career options and found her mother in their comfortable kitchen one day to ask her if nursing might not be a good career choice. Her mother had been a nurse and thought it was an admirable profession. Although Dorothy had not excelled at mathematics in high school because she found it uninteresting, she believed that she could work hard at her maths and sciences in an upgrading year and apply for nursing school. Her mother, always busy doing something around the house or knitting for her two daughters and husband, was ironing some clothes in the kitchen.

Without really looking up, Mrs. Ley talked about her cousin, Dr. Jessie McGeachy, who was then one of only a handful of women physicians in Toronto. Mrs. Ley suggested that Dorothy go pay her a visit. Dr. McGeachy encouraged Dorothy to consider a career in medicine and that meeting led Dorothy into a remedial year of math and science studies before entering medical school. During the War there was an opportunity for more women (10% of enrolment) to enter medical school as many of the male students had gone off to war. Ironically, when the war ended, those male students had precedent over the other students to complete their medical studies so that Dorothy had to wait an extra two years to complete her degree in 1948.

During her first year, Dorothy almost failed to pass because of her difficulties with mathematics. Never one to accept failure, she hired a tutor and worked extra hard to understand the challenging concepts of algebra, calculus and geometry. She passed that year and excelled in this subject in her following years.

The delay in her studies caused by the war led to some financial difficulties. Medical school was costly even then and she had promised her parents that she would pay her own way. She was fiercely independent, as was expected of her, but recognized that she could not complete her training without her father's financial help. Her father had not been pleased with Dorothy's decision to go into medical school. As was common for his generation, he believed that young women should not be exposed to the conditions that doctors witnessed in their daily practices. The Dean of Medicine had similarly advised her against medicine since he believed that Dorothy would only get married one day and quit medicine.

Dorothy went reluctantly to her father with a detailed accounting of what she would need to complete her studies with not a penny extra for the things someone in her early twenties might like to buy for herself. Mr. Ley examined Dorothy's itemized budget and agreed to loan her the funds she needed – to the exact penny she requested. Years later, after Mr. Ley had died, Dorothy found newspaper clippings of her success in her father's wallet. He was evidently very proud of his daughter.

During her studies, Dorothy developed an interest in diseases of the blood which led to her further studies in the area. She had begun her five-year post-graduate studies in obstetrics and gynaecology but her year of research at Toronto General Hospital under world-famous pathological chemist Dr. James Dauphinee convinced her that her interests lay in blood diseases. These studies resulted in her specializing in internal medicine with a sub-speciality in haematology. This was in 1950 before the time that cancer would have its own speciality, oncology.

When looking at someone's background it is important to understand what motivates their efforts. Dorothy's underlying motivation was similar to many people of her generation. Her motivation, shared by so many people of pre-war protestant Toronto, was commonly summarized as "worship God, serve mankind." She worked hard, took advantage of opportunities and difficulties that presented themselves and concentrated on her basic Christian principles. There was no single motivator, however, in her life. There was no life-defining event that encouraged her to pursue medicine, business, or palliative care.

In today's utilitarian, modern view of people as economic units within a global economy, it is hard to believe that people actually based their life's work on such simple words as "worship God, serve mankind." Simple words are not easily translated into daily living, however. There were choices in Dorothy's life about career, marriage and community service that would have dramatically altered her life. She based her decisions, however, on a strict code of right and wrong and would not accept second best for convenience sake.

Evidence of Dorothy's determination to serve mankind in the best ways she could is seen during her continuing medical studies. She chose a field that was new and untried but potentially rewarding if cures could be found for some of the blood diseases she was studying. She needed to travel beyond Toronto to learn as much as she could so she continued her studies at Barnes Hospital and the University of Washington in St. Louis before returning to Canada to practice haematology. She had an active practice (14-hour days), completed a further degree in pathological chemistry, taught at the University of Toronto, became the first woman head of a medical department (haematology and oncology) at Toronto Western Hospital and she continued to do research in the field. Later in her career she opened and operated fourteen testing laboratories which she later sold to MDS Labs. Not surprisingly, she became highly regarded by her medical peers becoming the first woman to receive an honourary fellowship of the American College of Physicians, and the first Canadian woman physician to receive the Canadian Medical Association Medal of Service.

Her proudest moment, however, came in the late 1960s when she presented a paper based on research she had done with colleagues in her field. The conference was in Stockholm and the occasion was so special to her because her mother, who had always supported her career choice, took her maiden airplane flight to hear, for the first time, her daughter speak in public. Her mother could not understand the content of the presentation but she did share in her daughter's success. That success had begun 20 years before in their kitchen discussion about going to nursing or medical school.

Dorothy's sense of right and wrong came from her parents and her parents' generation work ethic. Her father, of medium height and a strongly built man with an engineering degree was her role model. He had been a millionaire in Alberta before the stock market crash. Afterwards, he managed a foundry in Toronto and lived a comfortable upper-class existence in a beautiful neighbourhood in Toronto and always drove a Cadillac. She adored him as a child and followed his practice of demanding perfection of herself and of others. He was the most just man she ever knew and she tried to apply his sense of justice and fairness in her work and in her relationships.

Her mother, a diminutive, strong-minded Scots woman, held the family together with her intuitive abilities and skills. When Dorothy was younger she was convinced that her mother didn't understand her. It was only after becoming an adult that Dorothy realized her mother knew her better than she knew herself. Dorothy's mother lost most of her hearing while Dorothy was still a very young girl. People did not make a big fuss about such a disability in those days and everyone accommodated Mrs. Ley as a natural part of life.

Dorothy helped both of her parents to live at home until they died. Her father died in 1955 and her mother in 1971. Dorothy lived with her mother and her mother's cousin, Donalda (Donnie)

McGeachy until her mother moved back to her home town of Almonte, in the Ottawa Valley, to be with her older family members and friends.

Dorothy continued to live with her cousin until Donnie died in 1990. They had lived together for 39 years and were each other's best friends, confidantes and supporters. It was Donnie, for example, who convinced Dorothy to allow a group of people in Etobicoke, Ontario where they had lived for many years, to name a community hospice the Dorothy Ley Hospice. Dorothy hadn't liked the idea. She thought that such honours should be given to others more deserving than her and, perhaps, in honour of someone who had died. Donnie convinced her that she was the right person and encouraged her to help this group develop their program and services to meet the needs of their old community. It took many meetings over several years to finalize the approach this new community hospice would take and Dorothy was regularly involved to help them understand the hospice care philosophy and how it applied to community, versus hospital, based services. Dorothy understood these differences from her work in hospitals, her work with the Palliative Care Foundation, her efforts on the Board of Toronto's Casey House (a free-standing hospice for people with AIDS) and her own experiences helping people live at home until they died.

Donnie had a wonderfully full life as well. She had been an actress on the New York stage, a registered nurse and later one of the first licensed speech therapists in Canada. She helped develop the Speech-Language Pathology Program at the University of Toronto. She was a leader in her field and well known within the social circles of Toronto.

After Dorothy retired, they moved to Beaverton, Ontario on the shore of Lake Simcoe. They called their home "Tir N'an Og" which means "Land of Dreams" in Gaelic. From this home, Dorothy continued her retirement work in palliative care, including her time as Founder and President of The Palliative Care Foundation. She also became more involved in her church and the work of the Anglican Church in Ontario.

Many things have been said about Dorothy. Her friends and family have seen the Dorothy develop who was always an "easy touch" for help of any kind. The loyalty of her circle of family and friends speaks to the dedication and commitment that Dorothy had shown them. Her patients knew they could call her day or night, weekday or weekend for medical care and reassurance. She involved her patients in making decisions about their care to the point where she even gave some of them medical journals discussing the pros and cons of certain new treatments. She began using increasing doses of narcotics to manage pain long before palliative care was a reality in Canada. The RCMP were regular visitors to her office to monitor her use of narcotics, and they too became allies in providing the kind of care her patients needed.

Professionally, her work was demanding and so was she; she did not suffer fools lightly nor did she accept peers, leaders and others who did practice the palliative care philosophy faithfully. Her language was sometimes colourful and most often direct. Although she was shy and non-assertive by nature, excellence was her guide post and her public image of the assertive, elegant and forthright professional came out of her convictions.

Dorothy had experienced life as a patient when she was a child and her sister had pushed her off a dock. She broke her back during this accident and spent some time in a wheelchair and went through rehabilitation therapy. She continued to have back problems throughout her life and used the experience to try and understand what her patients were going through. For example, she learned from her own disability that a few minutes sitting down with a patient is worth a great deal more in comfort and concern than standing and looking down toward the patient as most physicians do.

Dorothy's life was full and varied. She was a licensed lay reader in the Anglican Church and her faith sustained her through many difficult and rewarding times during her life. She was a church organist for a time and gave sermons including some on the care of people who were dying and those living with AIDS. Her religion, however, did not prevent her from dealing with the practical nature of the political worlds of medicine and palliative care. In fact, her religious and spiritual beliefs provided the foundation for role modelling an inclusive model of care.

Dorothy's favourite stores to shop at were Canadian Tire and Aikenheads. She loved projects and thoroughly enjoyed buying the "toys" that allowed her to add on a study to her home, fix floors, mow her lawn with the latest mower, plant her garden with thousands of flowers, mend fences or survey the lake at the back of her home with one of her boats. Two of her closest friends helped out with the upkeep of her home and garden and they enjoyed sipping coffee with her while working on the garden or her home. Along with her projects she was a collector. She collected wood-carved ducks, stamps, first-day covers, non-fiction books and music.

Dorothy was as comfortable at a meeting of her peers to discuss policy and future needs in medicine as she was walking and working bare-foot in her garden. She could talk about any subject with ease because of her wide interests and her unsatiable love of reading and learning. She read only non-fiction works in medicine and the sciences, history, geography, philosophy, psychology, etc. She read novels only on airplane trips finishing the novel before leaving the plane and usually giving the book away to another passenger. She could talk sports (football was her favourite, followed by hockey, which she played in college as her team's goalie). Her private life was private which encouraged people to confide in her since they knew she did not discuss with others what was said to her privately.

One of her great passions were the dogs that she and Donnie had. Her favourite dog was a Cairn Terrier named Hamish and during the last years of her life she was comforted by Donnie's dog Sheena, a Lhasa Apsos.

Children of her closest friends called her Auntie Do and they knew they had a friend and advocate in Dorothy. She was not overtly demonstrative but she was always there with a smile, an ear to listen to all their excitement and a word of advice. Although she was always busy working on some report, going to meetings or preparing a presentation or article, she always took the time needed to help someone she knew without making them feel rushed. People would call her for medical advice or for tips on how to deal with the local government (she had been President of her local Ratepayers Association in Beaverton). She quietly helped people find work by making a phone call or two. She helped people find the right doctor for the right treatments and gave suggestions about what her friends might ask for in the way of support. She found pleasure in her friends, home, work and more than the occasional New York Cherry Cheesecake or chocolate ice cream.

Politically she was small "c" conservative and liked the stability that the monarchy provided the Commonwealth. She felt she was always treated fairly by men and did not believe that women's lib helped women as much as they thought. Men and women worked well together when they both worked hard for a common purpose.

Perhaps one of the most difficult, yet rewarding, times of Dorothy's life was when she took care of Donnie in their home. Dorothy was a physician by profession and knew very little about the nursing skills required to take care of an ill person at home. Dorothy turned to a friend, Barbara McGeachy, a nurse, for guidance. Barbara taught Dorothy the nursing skills necessary to take care of Donnie. Dorothy learned to do everything and anything necessary and did them "as well as any nurse" (high praise from a nurse to a doctor). At first Dorothy was not sure if she could do it on her own but she became expert during the four to five months that Donnie was at home. When Dorothy needed to be away for some palliative care work, Barbara would come from Kingston to help out.

Donnie died a peaceful death at Tir N'an Og with the help of Dorothy and many friends who provided extra support and encouragement. Dorothy learned several things about providing palliative care in the home and used her experience to continue to teach palliative care to others.

At the beginning and ending of this book are testimonials by some of the people who worked with Dorothy over the years. Their comments speak for themselves. How will Dorothy's closest friends remember her? When I asked them that question during individual interviews there was a consistency in their replies.

They will remember Dorothy as a caring, compassionate healer of people's bodies, minds, and even souls. She was action oriented and wanted to see results. She had will power that was extraordinary. When she made her mind up about something, which might take quite some time to accomplish, she never wavered from her decision and always followed throughout regardless of the personal cost to her. As one friend noted, "She showed more courage than anyone I've ever seen in their last months of life. She never complained, never asked 'Why me,' was never bitter that she didn't live as long as others, and never complained about pain or discomfort."

She was honest and direct with her friends who asked for advice. She knew instinctively when something was wrong with someone and would call or write them offering help, encouragement or support. She showed up on people's doorsteps at just the right time when someone needed her.

Others remember her quiet elegance and dedication. They remember that she was giving a keynote address at a conference one time after recent surgery related to her cancer. She always kept her commitments regardless of her own personal situation so she gave the address without comment about her recent surgery. After the presentation, she asked two of her friends at the conference, who were nurses, to help her change her medical dressings in her hotel room. No one else ever knew, and more importantly, no one else needed to know according to Dorothy. She did not want pity nor the image of a martyr or hero.

How would Dorothy like to be remembered? Again, her friends had some thoughts. They agreed that Dorothy would like to be remembered as a compassionate physician who practiced excellence for the whole person rather than concentrate on their disease. She was a mentor to so many people in the field of oncology and palliative care and she was proud of that teaching role. She was a loyal friend who encouraged others to reach beyond their comforts to achieve their very best. She criticized programs and protocols rather than people and wanted to act as a role-model for others in providing the palliative care philosophy of care.

In a sentence, Dorothy wanted to be remembered as an "old fashioned" doctor who took care of the patient and the family, combining physical, emotional and spiritual support. She was down to earth. Her awards, accomplishments were not a big deal to her. She just did those things that were important to her regardless of the rewards. She would not want to be remembered as someone above the rest of us but as an ordinary, hard-working person who used her abilities in the best possible way and worked hard to improve everything she did. As one friend concluded, "She would be embarrassed by all the fuss made to her in tributes."

Palliative Care: Past, Present & Future

The medieval hospices – whether the great fortress-hospital of St. John at Rhodes, the elegant hospice in the French town Beaune, or the myriad of small hospices associated with monasteries throughout Europe – were dedicated to the physical and spiritual care of the sick and the dying, and the Christian burial of the dead. Whether the traveller was a knight on the journey to Jerusalem, or a poor beggar on the journey of life, the ancient hospices were way stations, resting places, a place of care and concern for both the body and the spirit. These people were called "My Lords the Sick" and that is how they were treated.

But the world changed. Society changed. With the waning of monastic influence and changing social patterns, the number of hospices in the old sense decreased. A different pattern of care developed – the hospital. Gradually, with the advent of the Industrial Revolution, our western society increasingly valued order, efficiency and social discipline and came to regard a human being as an economic unit. "My Lords the Sick" became an admitting number and a disease code on a chart. Modern health care became the repository of those who were unable to contribute to an industrialized, super achieving society or a place to repair its damaged tools and get people back to the work place. The repository health facilities we call nursing homes (an oxymoron) or chronic care hospitals. The repair facilities we call hospitals or health science centres.

Palliative care has certain fundamental characteristics that set it apart from this industrialized, high-technology care we ordinarily provide to sick people. In the first place, palliative care is provided to people who are terminally ill, whose care is aimed not at curing a disease but at improving the quality of their life of someone who is dying. Dame Cicely Saunders, the British founder of the modern hospice movement said, that hospice care is there to make it possible for people who are dying to live fully until they die.

Death is not a disease. The process of dying is not a clinical diagnosis. People who practice palliative care must be aware of the differences between a patient and a terminally ill person. In the acute care system, patients of necessity give up their autonomy, their decision-making power, to their caregivers. People in hospice should be able to take back that power. They, and only they, should have the right to choose the nature of the care they will receive and where it will be given. And, dare I venture, when it will be stopped. Freedom of choice not to receive any more aggressive treatment that attempts to cure an illness or the choice not to use a ventilator or receive artificial feedings must be an integral part of any palliative care program – and it must extend from the patient to include family and friends. Freedom of choice, however, does not extend to the so called right to chose assisted suicide or euthanasia as these practices will certainly lead to the deaths of vulnerable people in our society.

Apart from the underlying philosophy, what is it that makes palliative care unique? Cicely Saunders laid down the essentials for a program over twenty years ago. They have not changed. First, a skilled interdisciplinary team – not just multidisciplinary, but interdisciplinary. There is a great difference. We tend in health care to put people from different disciplines in a room and tell them they are a team. In reality, all they are is a multidisciplinary group.

In general, we have failed to teach health care professionals team dynamics, to make them understand the different nature of leadership in an interdisciplinary setting. One of the great strengths of palliative care is the concept of the interdisciplinary team. No one person can provide palliative care. Every member of the team is equal, and "the team" includes the person who is dying, their family, and every person involved in their care, from volunteers to housekeeping staff, home support people and doctors and nurses. Each one is equally important.

At present, not all people who practice hospice care share that same palliative care philosophy. We come from different backgrounds and with different basic assumptions about how to value life. The patient-centred palliative care philosophy is broad enough to encompass most religious and fundamental beliefs. Therefore, until we share the same palliative care philosophy, we will continue to repeat the communication and treatment errors of the past decades. Interdisciplinary team work and a common philosophic base are required for successful hospice care and must become a priority for all hospice programs. To those well on the road to this realistic goal, they need to continually renew their commitment to their common philosophy and team approach, especially as new members join the team. For those programs still grappling with these questions, their priority must begin with these basics – immediately.

Pain and symptom control is one of the major components of palliative care. Without it, the rest is rhetoric. It is impossible to counsel dying persons if they are in pain. We now have the knowledge and the drugs, for example, to manage physical cancer pain and most symptoms. Unfortunately 90% of people admitted to hospice programs are admitted because of mismanaged cancer pain. Why? In my opinion, it is in part because of the attitude of doctors and nurses (and to a certain extent of patients) that people with cancer have pain and little can be done about it. I have heard this expressed by home care nurses and physicians in the last six months! In part too, it is because good pain and symptom management requires time and painstaking attention to detail. It cannot be done with "standing orders." Time, in our modern health care system, is a scarce commodity. It should be said, however, that pain and symptom control has improved in the past decade. There is a growing awareness of new drugs, new techniques, improved methods of management. There is a growing willingness to find the time.

There is also a growing awareness that our skills at managing pain and symptoms for people with cancer, and more recently for people living with AIDS and amyotrophic lateral sclerosis (ALS), should be extended and expanded to all people with a terminal or life-threatening illness.

Accepting the patient and family as the unit of care can make care very untidy. Not all families either want to be, or can be, part of care. An increasing number of people live alone. Family economics may make it impossible for family involvement. Not all patients want their families to be involved. And yet this, like the interdisciplinary team, is one of the great strengths of palliative care. It shifts the focus from a patient with a terminal illness to a person who is part of a dynamic, ongoing life situation – that will continue after their death. With patient and family as the centre of care we can never become complacent in believing we are meeting all the needs of all those we care for. At best, we provide them a safe, comfortable environment where they have the control to live out their last days as they see fit.

Palliative care, or hospice care as it is also called, began in Canada in hospitals. It is said of Canadians that we are the most institutionalized society in the world and that if we don't have a purpose-built institution for a new idea we will design and build one. To a degree this has coloured our perception of what constitutes such care. In Canada, we have emphasized institutional care to the detriment of community care. The result has been that community care in all its aspects has been neglected, or at best, provided as an interim measure or as a temporary adjunct to institutional care – not as an alternative. As well, we have tended to transfer the institutional model into the community setting without giving too much thought to the impact of that transfer on the community in which it is given.

The institutional model continues to be a major driving force of palliative care in Canada because that is where many of the professional leaders of palliative care still work. Are we really talking about palliative care when we talk about beds and units and cost-benefit analysis and institutions? Are we not forgetting the basic definition of palliative care? Our acute care institutions were designed, built and staffed to practice acute care medicine. Our entire health care delivery systems has been designed to do just that. In the face of changing patterns of demography, public expectations and government funding we seem to be trying to force new functions into old forms.

Our chronic care institutions, for example, are acute care institutions modified for another use. We even talk about extended care! Extended from what? We can no longer allow ourselves the luxury of developing palliative care programs for patients who are terminally ill of malignant disease alone. This country and the rest of the Western world is faced with the phenomenon of a rapidly increasing elderly population.

I have some real concern that palliative care will remain a WASP (White Anglo-Saxon Protestant) middle class phenomenon paid for by government insurance and limited mostly to people with cancer and AIDS. Who will help those who have other terminal or life- threatening illnesses? Where are the visible minorities in palliative care? Who represents the needs of other religious groups? Who represents the views of poorer, marginalized Canadians who are dying?

So far we have been content, and we have been able, to institutionalize a high percentage of the elderly in our population. We

Part I

The introduction and two chapters of Part I were written by Dorothy Ley and are taken from parts of her speeches, articles, and interviews.

Introduction:

Straight from the Heart

by Dorothy Ley

> And because right is right,
> To follow right
> Is wisdom in the scorn of consequence.
>
> **Anonymous**

Palliative care is about living and the meaning of life. It's about loss and grief and joy. It's about giving and receiving. It's about caring and sharing. It's about tears and laughter. These short words may sound trite but they are not. They are very powerful words when acted upon. In short, palliative care is about life, not death. We must always remember that.

Palliative care is a philosophy of care, not a particular kind of health care. It is rooted in hospice, a thread that goes back to a dusty road in Galilee and the story of the Good Samaritan. It is founded on the principle that we are our brother's keeper. Both Christian religion and spiritual care have been at the heart of hospice from its beginnings in the fourth century A.D. when the monk Fabiola established a hospice in pagan Rome for Christian pilgrims from Africa. The tradition of the medieval Knights Hospitaller was based on the injunction of Christ in the 25th Chapter of the Gospel according to St. Matthew, "Inasmuch as you have done it unto one of the least of these, my brethren, you have done it unto Me."

have been accused of warehousing them. There is a growing feeling that such treatment is no longer acceptable. It is not economically acceptable and it is becoming increasingly less acceptable socially. The elderly population in the year 2000 will be better educated, better travelled, more socially aware and less likely to be passive about their care than the preceding generations. It is absolutely essential in our future management of the elderly, and the incurably ill as well as the terminally ill, that we apply the philosophy and principles of palliative care to provide people with the physical, emotional, spiritual and informational supports they need.

The institutionally-based mind set has inhibited our ability to provide for the full development of active integrated home care in palliative care, although this should be where the greatest emphasis is placed. It is interesting that surveys of Canadian palliative care programs in 1986 and 1990 revealed a dramatic increase in community-based activity with little change in hospital programs. The emphasis in the community has been on independent and volunteer-driven programs, although in 1990 there was an increase in those associated with community agencies and an associated increase in the professional components. The present thrust in Ontario towards the provision of community based, long-term care, coupled with a decrease in hospital beds may well provide the impetus necessary to the development of a balanced, integrated palliative care system. Who knows? Success may come from adversity.

If one accepts the principle that the patient and family are the unit of care, then it follows naturally that palliative care is for the family too. There is a tendency, once a person dies, to pause in remembrance and then get on to the next person who needs care. The family is still there, still our responsibility, still has its needs for care. Every palliative care program must build into itself active bereavement follow-up. Every bereaved person, no matter how strong, how balanced, how well supported, needs to know that the people who cared for the person they loved remember them in their grief and their loss. It may only be a phone call or a card or a brief visit, but it is part of palliative care. In some 10% of the families, the team may recognize the need for professional support – and should be able to initiate it.

No matter the setting (home, hospital, free-standing hospice) the same kind of care and the same quality of care must be provided.

There may be special skills or special team members required for different settings but the care must be the same. The patient and family should have a choice of care and of setting. Whether such choice is limited by government or professional fiat or by lack of facilities, the end result is the same – it is impossible to provide good palliative care without freedom of choice. Unfortunately, in most of Canada, that choice does not exist. It must be the goal of all who work in palliative care to create a system in which it does exist.

How does one create an ideal system of palliative care? One of the main methods of creating ideal palliative care is to return to the philosophy of providing physical, emotional, spiritual and informational supports. We have done quite well at providing physical and emotional supports to those people lucky enough to receive formal palliative care but we have only paid lip service in many cases to providing good spiritual care. We lack a coherent value base from which to provide such care and that is why so many programs are going into directions that hospice care was never intended to go. Ideally hospice programs should be small to meet the individual needs of people who are ill and their families. We should minimize the professionalization of the natural, compassionate care that is palliative care. We are concentrating so much on policies, procedures, funding formulas, and government involvement that we are losing sight of why hospice began and who we, as care providers, are in business to serve. We are shifting to a model of care where our loyalties are with the system of care (regardless of the organization) rather than with the person who is dying. These are grave problems demanding immediate attention and resolution.

What are the barriers to a palliative care system? Aside from our inconsistent approach to the palliative care philosophy, there are practical deficiencies that continue to face us in the 1990s. They have changed little from the 1980s and they include: too little professional staffing, too little integration of services and cooperation between programs and facilities, insufficient education for professional and volunteer staff, incomplete practical standards of care, and insufficient, ongoing funding.

One can focus on any one of these and make a good argument for its importance. To me, however, the single greatest challenge is educating people.

There is a strong "death" education movement in both the

United States and Europe that believes that one starts in the school system to change attitudes towards death and dying. The International Work Group on Death and Dying and Bereavement has developed assumptions and principles concerning death education that address our society's prejudices and fears concerning death. They should be mandatory reading for everyone in palliative care (see Appendix). The ability to provide good palliative care is affected by society's attitude – which is mirrored in the attitude of our patients and their families.

No system of palliative care can develop without educated professionals. At present we do not teach medical students, nurses or other health and social care professionals the principles of palliative care at the undergraduate level except in a spotty fashion. There is almost no classroom teaching and very little clinical experience provided. Some universities are beginning to take tentative steps to correct this. There is now a chair in palliative medicine at the University of Calgary, the University of Ottawa and I believe at Memorial University of Newfoundland in St. John's. There is a well-developed palliative care program at Dalhousie University and an excellent one in the University of Victoria – and a superb one at McMaster University in Hamilton. At the University of Toronto, the family practice training program is providing clinical and classroom experience for some of its interns, both at Mount Sinai Hospital and in the community.

But education is more than teaching doctors and nurses pain and symptom management and the concept of total pain with all its physical, psychological and emotional aspects. It is teaching all members of the team the principles we have just discussed. It is accepting volunteers as active, educated members of the team and providing them with standardized training. It is teaching health care professionals team dynamics where everyone shares in the decision-making and responsibilities of the team. It is teaching them how to counsel and when not to. It is demonstrating hand-holding or not doing anything at all. It is teaching them that case conferences are not just reviewing care plans! It is giving them attitudes that will last their professional lifetimes, whether they become high tech experts or family physicians. It is, in fact, changing the way they view the people for whom they care. Building on that is the need to create teachers and researchers and specialists in palliative care who will educate the next generation.

What are the basic components of palliative care? The basic foundation of care in 1981 was pain and symptom control followed by counselling (emotional support) and spiritual care, if there was time. By this decade I have come to recognize that a more appropriate foundation is spiritual care followed by counselling and pain and symptom control. Pain and symptom control must come first in the practical application of palliative care but under the foundation and attitude of spiritual care. Spiritual care is what sets palliative care apart and gives it its unique characteristics.

Death is a spiritual event. Its nearness creates a desire to identify and strengthen what is of value in one's life. We want to tidy up the ends, to put first things first. To be unable to do so can generate a desolate feeling of meaningless. To me that is the essence of spiritual pain – to feel that one is meaningless or that one's life has had no meaning.

Viktor Frankl, the famed Vienna psychiatrist and survivor of Nazi concentration camps, has reminded us that each must find the meaning in their own life and that no one can tell another person what the meaning of his life should be. Our role as caregivers is to give people the opportunity and the time to work through and solve their own problems – to find their own meanings. We may need to be no more than a presence. The dying, as Cicely Saunders has said, "Ask only that we watch with them, that we be there." We can give them freedom and space by controlling their physical pain. We can walk beside them on their journey. We can understand them because of our own experiences, our own pain, our own mortality. The concept of the wounded healer is at the root of modern hospice care. We may not understand the specific feelings of someone who is dying but we have our own wounds, our own emotional difficulties and our own unresolved issues.

There are those who might think this is an unnecessary topic for discussion. After all, spiritual care runs through hospice care like a thread. It is one of the pillars of hospice, no matter where you put it – top or bottom. Or is it? Are we assuming that after the narcotics and the nursing, after the counselling and the initiation of bereavement follow-up, after the service on the hospice floor, spiritual care falls neatly into place on the chart – particularly if the chaplain has been involved in the final hours or days of care and has been able to talk to family and friends?

And so we go on our way to the next dying person. But 94% of American Hospice Programs surveyed by the Joint Commission on Hospital Accreditation failed to demonstrate adequate spiritual care – adequate address of people's need to find meaning in their life and in their dying. Although we consider spiritual care to be a fundamental component of palliative care only 58% of Canadian programs have a chaplain.

Spiritual care has been described as the last necessary required revolution in palliative care. One's concept of spirituality is both intimate and personal – and so it should be, no matter one's age, cultural or religious background. We are spiritual beings deep within ourselves and must bring that spirituality to palliative care. Even in our search for scientific excellence, in our creation of standards, our demands for formalized education and for government funding to provide a model system of care – we must never forget that we must reach out beyond our narrow interests – to reach out from our inner selves to the people for whom we care – all of them. For love is the litmus test of palliative care and spirituality is its heart.

Pillars of Care 1

by Dorothy Ley

Barter

Life has loveliness to sell
All beautiful and splendid things;
Blue waves whitened on a cliff,
Soaring fire that sways and sings,
And children's faces looking up
Holding wonder like a cup.

Life has loveliness to sell
Music like a curve of gold,
Scent of pine trees in the rain
Eyes that love you, arms that hold
And for your spirits still delight
Holy thoughts that star the night.

Spend all you have for loveliness.
Buy it and never count the cost.
For one white singing hour of peace
Count many a year of strife well lost.
And for a breath of ecstacy
Give all you have been, or could be.

Sara Teasdale

The basis of a good palliative care service involves meeting the physical, emotional, spiritual and informational needs of people who are dying and their families. This requires a skilled, interdisciplinary team of doctors, nurses, pharmacists, clergy, homecare staff, social workers, therapists, dieticians, homemakers, volunteers and others as needed. Most patients do not require the services of all these people. The ideal number is small and based on the expressed needs of the patient rather than the wishes of the team.

This team must be able to provide effective pain and symptom control with the patient and family as the unit of care and as active members of the team (if they choose). There must be an active, integrated home care system to allow most people to stay at home for as long as they like, including to live at home until their death. There must be bereavement follow-up with the underlying assumption that most people do not need bereavement therapy but recognition that someone important in their lives has died.

No palliative care program is effective without providing care for the caregivers. Caregivers go through many of the same physical and emotional ups and downs as family caregivers and they need similar supports. They need others to recognize when a special patient has died. They need to share their skills and knowledge but also their fears and concerns.

All of these components rest on the assumption that the patient has freedom of choice. Some patients may not want their pain and suffering relieved and their wishes must be accepted. They should always have the opportunity to change their mind but never by manipulation. Some patients may not want to resolve family issues and difficulties. Some patients may not even want you in the room with them. These are difficult situations for the caregivers but ones that must be addressed with respect for the patients' choices and with opportunities for them to understand the consequences of those decisions.

In the next four sections, we will look at these four pillars of care: physical, emotional and social, spiritual and informational.

1. Physical

There is no Death.
What seems so is transition.

Anonymous

There is growing expertise in the relief of physical pain and the management of symptoms to maintain activity and to provide a degree of independence and self-esteem. Nevertheless, many people continue to suffer unrelieved pain and poorly managed symptoms because of a lack of education and because of faulty attitudes on the part of health care professionals.

My purpose here is not to give a medical lecture on proper pain and symptom management. Books by Derek Doyle, Ivan Goldberg, Larry Librach, Cicely Saunders, and the Expert Advisory Committee on the Management of Severe Chronic Pain in Cancer Patients do an admirable job of this.

The key point to make here is that there is now good evidence that palliative care can relieve virtually all physical discomfort. The vast majority of people can be relatively pain-free and alert until hours or days before they die. People suffer needlessly in Canada at present. This is inexcusable. The knowledge and role models of excellent care are readily available. The notion that people must suffer pain is absurd. Until this simple fact is recognized and addressed, excellent palliative care will only remain possible for a small percentage of dying patients.

The process for managing pain is quite simple. Patients, family members and non-medical health care providers can understand the basics easily. What is required of the physician is careful attention to detail and an ability to listen closely to what the patient says. The physician must make a detailed assessment and take a complete history. When pain is moderate, the patient may receive medication such as aspirin. When the pain worsens, the physician prescribes a mild narcotic such as codeine. When the pain become intolerable, narcotics such as morphine are used. Basically these are the three levels of medications used to treat pain. Other medication may be necessary to deal with other symptoms (e.g. constipation, arthritic pain, a feeling of breathlessness) but for the pain resulting from the terminal illness these are basically the three steps.

The myth that too much pain medication will lead to addiction is just that – myth. When medication is used to combat pain, there is no "high" associated with its use and, therefore, no addiction. The oft-stated belief that too much narcotic medication results in a patient building up a tolerance to the drug is also untrue: patients survive years on very high dosages of narcotics that a few years ago were considered lethal. Our knowledge of the proper use of medications has resulted in safe and effective practices yet many health care providers and members of the general public alike still believe these myths.

What are the reasons for inadequate pain management? The biggest reason is the inadequate application of current skills and knowledge by physicians and other health care providers. People are not receiving sufficient medication in most cases. Others are not receiving the right medication at the right dose, at the right time and in the right way (usually orally or by suppository) resulting in too much pain or too much unnecessary sedation. The old method of waiting until the pain returned before giving more medication (called PRN – as required) is outdated and ineffective. There is also a failure to monitor changes in the patient's needs over time and to change the medication or dosage when necessary. There is a failure to use other drugs to work along side those being used to supplement the proper effects. Psychological conditions that ameliorate or intensify pain are inadequately identified and addressed. The consequences of dietary and cultural remedies are not adequately considered relative to the drug treatment being followed. There continues to be a large gap in the availability of pain management services throughout the country which isolates people from different geographic, ethnic, linguistic and financial backgrounds.

Pain management continues to be generalized for most patients rather than individualized to each person's needs, sensation of pain and illness. Physicians will write, and are taught to write, the same order for each patient with the same illness. You can go through charts and find the same prescription for all patients regardless of the patient's own perceptions and needs. Only if there is a noticeable difference, such as a patient weighing less than one hundred pounds, is there a change in the prescription. As well, many physicians continue to prescribe medication "prn", which means that the patient receives medication when their pain returns. Study after study has shown that the most effective pain management requires regular doses of appropriate medication so that the patient does not feel the pain returning.

There remain patients who have difficult pain management situations. However, there are always things one can do to minimize physical pain to tolerable levels using medications, TENS machines, radiation therapy, meditation or prayer, biofeedback, and even surgery. In only the rarest cases (most physicians would never encounter such a case) would it be necessary to anaesthetize a patient suffering extreme pain or discomfort.

Although pain and suffering are generally linked together in the minds of patients and physicians it is important they recognize the distinction between them. We must return to the concept of total pain: the physical, emotional, and spiritual pains that people feel. All pain is subjective and no one should be treated in exactly the same way as someone else with the same disease. Pain and symptom management must be approached on an individual basis and open to the effective use of both medical and non-medical treatments. Severe pain can be handled if a patient knows its cause, or believes that it can be relieved and that it will soon end. However, even minor pain can be magnified and cause suffering if its cause is unknown or believed to be life-threatening (such as cancer) or if its presence is a symptom of a hopeless condition.

Suffering on the other hand, may exist without any physical symptoms. It is related to one's "self" or personality and is experienced by "persons." People can suffer because of the illness or loss of a loved one or because they feel lost relative to the world or their relationships. People with a terminal illness suffer a series of losses. They vary from loss of physical form from surgery, treatment or disease to loss of freedom of movement, loss of control over their lives or family, financial or professional loss. Ultimately they are aware of the greatest loss of all – life itself.

The sense of loss, the feeling of being diminished as a person are aggravated by the symptoms of illness – pain, weakness, nausea, shortness of breath. Suffering occurs and continues as long as the patient perceives that there will be no end to the symptoms of illness and no relief from the series of losses.

The role of the physician and nurse is to reduce both the pain and the suffering. It is ironic that in their desire to relieve symptoms, physicians often aggravate suffering. We must learn to treat patients and not diseases, and set the goals of our treatment to fit their life situation. We must recognize that it is the quality and not necessarily the length of life that is important. The patient's fears of pain, choking to death, or increasing debilitation must be acknowledged and addressed with compassion and skills.

Hospice care was designed with the following concepts in mind: first to relieve pain and symptoms and provide physical comfort for the patient, in a way that will allow them to participate in the life around them, and secondly, to counsel and support the patients, their family and community, and to enhance their involvement in care. Finally, to provide the personal and spiritual counselling needed to maintain the integrity of that patient as a persons, to minimize and relieve their suffering. As Cicely Saunders puts it: "To help you to live until you die."

The other three pillars of care describe some of the ways to provide that support once physical pain and symptoms are relieved.

2. Emotional

Prayer for a Very New Angel

God, God, be lenient her first night there.
The crib she slept in was so near my bed;
Her blue and white wool blanket was so soft,
Her pillow hollowed so to fit her head.

Teach me that she'll not want small rooms or me.
When she has You and Heaven's immensity!

I always left a light out in the hall.
I hoped to make her fearless in the dark,
And yet, she was so small - one little light.
Not in the room, it scarcely mattered. Hark!

No, No; she seldom cried!
God, not too far for her to see,
This first night, light a star.

And in the morning, when she first woke up,
I always kissed her on her left cheek where,
The dimple was. And o, I wet the brush,
It made it easier to curl her hair.

Just, just tomorrow morning, God, I pray,
When she wakes up, do things for her my way!

V. A. Storey

Modern hospice care began in a white, Anglo-Saxon, Christian community in Great Britain. We now live and practice hospice care in a multicultural, pluralistic society. Each of us has our own orientation toward death and dying as a result of the ideas and attitudes of persons we associate with dying – the doctor, the nurse, the funeral director, or the man that drove the car that killed your friend.

This orientation is composed of places – hospitals (80% of North Americans die in hospitals and 90% of those wish they didn't). It is composed of things. What do we associate with death? The smell of lavender in a quiet bedroom in a beloved home, or, in my case, remembering my grandmother with her knitting needles and my grandfather with his pipe. Or do we remember intravenous tubes in an intensive care unit of a hospital? The death system is shaped by our experience of death. Our death systems are shaped as well by life expectancy. In Tanzania, for example, life expectancy is 48 years while in Canada it is 78. We think of death in our society in terms of old people in institutions. In Tanzania they think of death in terms of young people at home. The African lives within a village, within an extended family. We Westerners are isolated; trapped within a complex society. I am an individual. If I died tomorrow, I'm not certain that my death would make much impact on the world in which I lived. If I were an African and a grandmother, my death would make a tremendous difference on the world in which I lived.

A fundamental problem in palliative care as it becomes more international, more cross-cultural, is the tension that exists when we come to care for people with different death systems. Culture is a dominant force in determining health, illness and caring patterns for every society. It is essential to understand the health and illness beliefs of other cultures if we are to provide the holistic care that we espouse. The multi-cultural nature of modern society is reflected not only in the diversity of the recipients of care but the caregivers themselves.

How do you explain the needs of a Scottish-Canadian octogenarian to a 28-year old Sikh physician from the Punjab? Or for that matter, vice versa? In carrying out a cultural assessment there are two fundamental principles that should not be violated. Firstly, do not stereotype. Having said that, I know that all of us do stereotype people in order to make sense of our increasingly complex world. Since we stereotype by nature, the reasonable alternative is to find out if your stereotype is accurate. For example, people of Scottish and Dutch backgrounds have reputations for being very frugal in how they spend money or give gifts. If you are working with someone of this background, and it is relevant to your work, find out if this stereotype is accurate for this person. All members within any ethnic group are not identical.

Secondly, do not emphasize differences. Understand the important differences (for example, cultural/religious rituals performed at the time of death) but concentrate on the unique nature of any particular group.

The cultural mosaic affects all components of hospice care whether it be pain management, psycho-social or spiritual supports. In any assessment, there are three factors that must be considered: culture, language, and religion. To provide effective palliative care one must understand: the person's perception of death, health and illness, their tradition of care, the role of the family and community (if any), the perception of the caregivers involved, and the person's spirituality.

3. Spiritual

Theology

The blade is sharp, the reaper stout,
And every daisy dies.
Their souls fluttering about -
We call them butterflies.

Joyce Kilmer

It is crazy to believe that religion is the major motive behind providing palliative care. Spirituality, however, is a major factor. Dying and death are spiritual events. Providing spiritual support is not something that happens automatically within hospice, nor is it the sole responsibility of chaplains or clerics to provide spiritual support.

Modern society tends to compartmentalize care with spiritual care left to professionals. We constantly see charts of interdisciplinary teams with interconnected circles representing each team member and chaplaincy clearly marked as the department that provides spiritual care.

Each member of the hospice team has the capacity to provide spiritual care, although each person's perception of such care will be different. One's concept of spirituality is both intimate and personal–and so it should be. We are spiritual beings deep within ourselves. It is from that well that each must draw when caring for dying people.

Spirituality is commonly used to describe the differences that exist between mankind and other animals. The dictionary defines it as "that which concerns the spirit or higher or moral qualities, especially as regarded in a religious aspect." The concept of a spiritual soul is not found in the same way in Judaism or non-Western religions as it is in Christianity. To quote John Morgan (1988), "We who live in a Western culture shaped by both the language of the Greek intellectual experience and the Christian religious experience identify the idea of spirituality with religion."

A distinction must be made between religion and spirituality. Religion can be defined as an organized set of practices that surround a traditionally-defined belief in the existence of a God or divine, super-human, ruling power. Such practices are set down in sacred writings or declared by authoritative teachers. There are other definitions. Religion is, in some respects, a set of tools used to express or practice one's beliefs. Spirituality may be (and hopefully is) a part of religious beliefs or practices. However, religion may, or may not, be part of one's spirituality. Those with strong religious ties may have difficulty recognizing this fact.

Spirituality is our relationship with the infinite and, it should be added, with our fellows. It has been said that it integrates our identities. It is the essence of self. It is the I. It is the God within each of us, the part that can commune with the transcendent. It underlies our capacity to forgive, to create, to love and to accept love. It frequently is intensified by approaching death. Our spirituality is what we seek when we search for meaning in our lives.

In our industrialized, high-technology health care systems of today there is little room for caring for the whole person (mind, body and soul) and their families. The moral and ethical issues of our time (abortion, capital punishment, euthanasia, war) are those related to death. In medieval times, death was accepted as the completion of life, no matter how short, to be shared with family, friends and one's community. Over time it has come to be seen as a violent disruption of living, calling forth grief, a pervasive sense of loss and intense fear.

In the seventeenth century, in the midst of profound social change, Descartes put forward the concept of the dualism of mind and body. The Church assumed responsibility for the mind (and soul) and science (or medicine) for the body. This philosophy has had a profound and lasting effect on the practice of medicine and ultimately on both society's and medicine's attitude toward death and dying. Today we are still caught in the dichotomy that Descartes enunciated so long ago, the separation of mind and body. Scientific medicine became increasingly intrusive in the process of dying, so much so that Ivan Illich coined the phrase "the medicalization of death" to describe a society in which death had become faceless, secularized, institutionalized and robbed of its humanity. We developed the technical ability to keep people alive but we removed the humanity from death. Aries, a leading French scholar, subsequently wrote that the modern hospital was the only place where death could hide (1951).

In the twentieth century the scientific explosion of high technology and aggressive treatments to cure illness combined with rapid urbanization to isolate people from natural birth and death. When I was a child many of my family were farmers. I knew that people got old and couldn't farm and died. I knew that cats and dogs and other animals died. I knew that every year a cycle of birth and death took place. I was lucky because I grew up with an understanding of the place of death in my own world. I knew when I was practising that many of my patients did not have that understanding.

My childhood, as for all of us, coloured my attitude to death and dying. In my lifetime, the locus of care has shifted from the community, where my grandfather, grandmother and both my parents died, to "high tech" institutions. The role of the physician changed from a family friend and confidante to that of a distant, authoritative, scientific figure. The new technology and the increased availability of medical care as a result of universal or private health care insurance plans justified the public's belief that health was a right and fostered the illusion of medical infallibility and the indefinite deferment of death.

We became a death-denying society cared for by health professionals who saw the maintenance of life and not the quality of that life as a measure of competence and turned away from death as expression of failure. All of us caregivers bear some of the responsibility for creating that milieu. The stage was set for the modern hospice movement. Hospice, in the twentieth century, began as a revolt against medical attitudes and practices and the rigid institutional bureaucracy that reduced dying people to the state of a disease in a bed. Again, medical and other health care professions share the burden of this high tech approach to care.

The social revolution of the sixties rejected establishment power, including medical power, and in part led to the questioning of the validity of the Cartesian philosophy of separation of mind and body. Cicely Saunders, in Great Britain, developed the hospice as an alternative form of holistic care for people dying difficult deaths with cancer. Her hospice, St. Christopher's, began in 1967 and grew out of her medical and evangelical Christian experiences. St.

Christopher's is a Christian institution and people of all faiths and cultures are welcomed. Kubler-Ross, a psychiatrist in America, studied the questions and concerns of those who were dying and found that there were many questions that went unanswered by their health care professionals – either because they had no answers or they did not listen to the questions. She actively promoted the concept of dying at home, surrounded by family and friends. These two women said, "Look, people are people. We must put faces on the dying. We must help people become whole again." It was a return, philosophically at least, to the medieval perspective of dying. The modern version demands using the high tech means available to relieve pain and other symptoms but we must never forget that we are dealing with people – people who have physical needs, who have social needs, and who have spiritual needs. People who are part of a family and a community – and they need our care as well. Kubler-Ross said, "Not only can we not answer the questions of these people, we don't even hear them." Truly listening brings out the spirituality of the people we care for and our own spirituality. It is not surprising that there is a strong spiritual component to the philosophy of hospice as developed by these women. Spirituality was, and is, the heart of modern hospice care.

No discussion of spiritual care in hospice would be complete without a consideration of the concept of total pain and the meaning of suffering. Total pain is made up of different components: physical, psychological, social, emotional and spiritual. Pain embraces the whole person. Physical pain must be managed first. We have the knowledge and tools but we are reaching only a small percentage (less than 10%) of the people who need our help. In fact, last year a homecare nurse said to me that "we have to accept that 'palliatives' are going to die with pain." Her comments reveal an attitude of isolating terminally ill people with the label "palliatives" and an attitude shared by many patients that people with cancer are going to die in pain – a self-fulfilling prophecy.

If hospice is to care for the whole person, the family and community must be included. To relieve social pain and to provide spiritual support, the hospice caregiver must be able to recognize the needs of the family and community and help them to come to terms with those needs and their own fears. A fundamental principle of hospice is that the centre of care must be the person who is dying and that person's family. "No man is an island" wrote John Donne. We cannot live apart from our relationships with others. In modern society the "family" unit frequently differs from the so-called "nuclear family." The family may include close friends and may not include, by the patient's definition, their parents, siblings or lovers. Is the family anywhere near the patient? If they are, do they want to be involved at all? Do they recognize (or care about) the dying person's need for coming to terms with their life? So many people live alone. The hospice caregivers may have to become a surrogate family.

It may be necessary to re-establish communication with the person who is ill and their family; to assist in the process of reconciliation. In many families there is much reconciliation to be done; there is some in every family. The goal of hospice care is to facilitate, not mandate, that reconciliation and help people to tie up loose ends, to take their farewells. However, as Cicely Saunders has so wisely pointed out, this is "not just a salvage operation, but an original opportunity, a moment for creation" (1988).

When we care for persons who are dying we must find out who they are. Who is that person? What is their essential being? There is a tendency in modern society to think of ourselves in terms of what we do. We consider a person to be manifested in their work, their interests, their accomplishments, but a person is more than that. Who are we deep inside ourselves? What are our inner concerns, our values? How can we make sense of it all at the end? How can we find meaning in our living and in our dying? That surely is the spiritual dimension of a person – and that is what we must seek when we care for people near the end of their lives. For some, their religious values and practices provide deep support and allow them to come to terms with their lives. For them the chaplain in a program is an essential member of the team. Others may have no relationship to a religion, or may have a sense of guilt, or unease, or a feeling that they were never able to measure up to the expectations of their family, their church or their God. The sermons, the sacraments, and the services do not reach them. As hospice caregivers, we must reach them, whether we wear a collar backwards, wear a white coat or a nurses' cap, or a volunteer's smock or push a broom as a housekeeper. Death is a spiritual event. It generates a desire to identify what is valuable and true in one's life. We want to tidy up the ends, to put first things first. The inability to do so in a person's life may generate a desolate feeling of meaningless.

This is the essence of spiritual pain, to feel that one is meaningless or that one's life has been meaningless. In Viktor Frankl's book *Man's Search for Meaning* (1987), he writes that if there is no way out of suffering then we have a responsibility for our attitude toward that suffering. In *When Bad Things Happen to Good People* (1981), Harold Kushner, a rabbi and father whose son died of a terminal illness, makes much the same point, that the pain is the reason and out of the pain and suffering comes understanding; comes the answer. Kushner also reiterates (as Job learned) that God does not ask us to do things that he does not give us the strength to do.

Frankl reminds us that no one can tell another person what the meaning of their life should be. Sometimes we in hospice care tend to sermonize. It is tempting to preach but we do not have the right to tell dying people the meaning of their lives, only to help them find it. The key to spiritual care is to give them the opportunity and the time to work through and solve their problems–to find their own meaning. We may need to be no more than a presence–to be there. As Saunders has remarked, there is a striking analogy between hospice care and Gethsemane. Christ was asking for meaning in what He had to do. He was asking that it not happen, but that if it did, He would be able to endure the pain and suffering that He knew lay ahead. How often our patients say to us, "I know I'm dying, I don't want to die and I don't want to be in pain, but if you help me I can do it. Just be here and help me." As Christ said to the disciples, "Could you not watch with me one hour?", so often we are asked, "Watch with me." One cannot die for another or grant them a good death. One can never walk in a dying person's shoes. It is their death. All we can do is walk beside them. Spiritual care is helping them to find the way to acceptance and peace.

Henry Nouwen, priest, writer and member of Jean Vanier's L'Arche communities wrote (1972) about the concept of the wounded healer, which is very important to hospice care. We understand because we too are wounded, because we too have pain. We understand because of who we are and because we have come to accept our own mortality. We must dig down deep inside and integrate the scattered parts of ourselves in order to be able to respond, even imperfectly, to a dying person's needs.

How do we help others? We caregivers are so diverse. We come from different backgrounds, from different beliefs, from different religions or no religion at all, and we are not dying. It is said that no one can imagine their own death. This means that when we care for dying people we cannot imagine what they are experiencing. However, we too can feel suffering. We can feel pain. We can feel loss. What can we do?

We can give them freedom and space by controlling their pain. We can listen. We may not have the answers, but we can listen. We can listen in such a way that we help them to find their own answers, and the gift of listening belongs to everyone on the team.

What is suffering? There are many definitions. Eric Cassel, an eminent scholar on the nature of suffering, has written eloquently about it and has focused new attention on the interrelationship between pain and suffering (1982). We suffer when we perceive an impending threat to our personality, to our personhood. Suffering is unique. Only humans can suffer. Furthermore, we can suffer for others. We suffer until the threat to our personhood is removed or until we can come to terms with it. Recognizing suffering and helping people to deal with suffering is part of spiritual care. Part of the ability to recognize suffering as distinct from pain lies in overcoming the concept of the dichotomy between mind and body.

Spirituality is implicit in the grieving process. If we, as hospice caregivers, accept the premise that our responsibility for care encompasses both patient and family, then our spiritual care must extend into the period of bereavement and include all those who grieve. The pain of grief is as real as the pain of cancer and, as in the management of physical pain, hospice care holds out the promise of relief. The bereaved, too, search for meaning in their loss and in the face of death. Like the dying, they need our skills, our compassion and the sense that we are there. Spiritual care should lead to the opportunity for both personal and community growth. To quote Delton Glebe, "The spirituality of pain is the healing that is hidden in the hurting" (1990).

There are a number of issues that affect spiritual care in modern society. There are global reasons, for example, for the current awareness of the need for spiritual care. R. J. Lifton makes some interesting and challenging comments in his book, *The Broken Connection* (1979). He reminds us that our sense of immortality depends on the link between life and death. In modern society our concept of that link has often been destroyed, for example, by nuclear war. We think of our immortality in terms of the world we leave behind. If there will be no world, how then do we conceptualize immortality.

The world has been struck recently with a series of natural disasters, in which thousands of people have perished. Chernobyl faced the world with sudden, insidious death over which there was no control. It could not be anticipated, could not be seen and struck silently thousands of miles from its source. It reinforced the world's sense of vulnerability. The death of seven astronauts was witnessed on television by millions of viewers. It, too, threatened our sense of control and shook our faith in science. There is a growing tendency at this time to question science and technology, and an increased impetus to examine the meaning of our lives.

AIDS is a world-wide pandemic that has generated a sense of fear and hopelessness and an increasing perception of man's helplessness and human frailty. Organized religion in the Western world has not been at the forefront of care for people with AIDS or their family and friends. In part this has been because AIDS first appeared in two marginalized groups in society – homosexuals and drug abusers – that the modern church, both theologically and spiritually, has difficulty accepting. The developing world on the other hand – particularly Africa – has been, and continues to be, devastated by a pandemic of HIV infection that has the potential for destroying the fragile economy of many countries and wiping out the first generation of people with modern education. The face of AIDS is clearly visible in Africa. It is the face of ignorance, of disease, of poverty and promiscuity, of social dislocation and changing lifestyle. The Western world, faced with escalating infection of women and children and rapid spread of HIV in the community, only now is beginning to recognize the true nature of this pandemic. Only now are we beginning to look at the broader problems underlying the spread of this virus – problems that are directly related to the spiritual values of modern society.

We still must care for those people in our society who are infected with HIV and who have AIDS. Hospice caregivers not only require special medical and nursing skills to care for terminally ill AIDS patients, but they must learn new counselling skills for people and communities that they may not understand. Traditionally, caregivers have been white and middle class. AIDS should be a stimulus to an increase in the numbers of homosexuals and lesbians and visible minorities who are active in hospice care. The ability to provide spiritual care depends on the recognition of the nature of the spirituality of others, although it may differ from ours. Those of us who profess to be Christian must examine the ways in which we treat both our fellow Christians and others. AIDS is calling on the church to examine its role in providing pastoral care for people who are infected with HIV, their families and friends, and pastoral care for caregivers who become infected. AIDS is calling the church to look at itself in a way it has not done for centuries.

Another issue facing hospice and spiritual care in hospice is the rapid increase in the number of elderly, especially the frail elderly, in North American society. By the year 2000 there will have been a 130 percent increase in the number of people over 85 since 1980. Over 70 percent of the people in hospice care are over 65 years old. We live in a competitive and materialistic society that puts a premium on dominance and power. Our perception of aging is one of decline in productivity and potential and increasing dependency and powerlessness. As caregivers we must resist the temptation to practice benign paternalism. There may be a gap of two or three generations between the dying elderly person and their caregivers. To provide spiritual care for the terminally ill elderly we must recognize the real nature of the person who is dying, the poignancy of their losses, the uniqueness of their perception of spirituality and their relationship to their religions. The elderly are more concerned about the quality of their lives than the length. They are frequently afraid of being abandoned physically, emotionally and spiritually. Hospice must find a way to reinforce their personhood and give them back the control that we so easily take away from them.

There are problems facing spiritual care in hospice that are associated with ethnic differences. I have examined some of the social issues regarding ethnic differences in the previous chapter including our different orientations to death and dying depending on our culture and backgrounds. Spiritual care and the differences and similarities of our spiritual backgrounds is not often discussed in palliative care in a practical way.

We try to care for people from different ethnic and religious backgrounds and we, the people who provide care, come from differing beliefs and have different spiritual concepts. There is compassion and concern in the Buddhist teaching. There is compassion and concern in the Jewish faith. Humanists are concerned with social justice and ethics, compassion and abiding commitment. All can, and do, provide spiritual care in hospice – and not only to their own. Indeed, we could, and should, develop ecumenical spiritual care in hospice.

Spiritual care has been described as the "unfinished revolution in palliative care" (Corless, 1986). Spirituality is difficult to describe and even more difficult to define. Norman Cousins stated the problem facing hospice care most eloquently in his book *The Anatomy of An Illness* (1979), "Death is not the ultimate tragedy of life. The ultimate tragedy is de-personalization – dying in an alien and sterile area, separated from the spiritual nourishment that comes from being able to reach out to a loving hand, separated from a desire to experience the things that make life worth living. Separated from hope."

In answer to the cry of the spirit, hospice says: We are here. We will be with you in your living and your dying. We will free you from pain and give you the freedom to find your own meaning in your own life – your way. We will comfort you and those you love–not always with words, often with a touch or a glance. We will bring you hope–not for tomorrow but for this day. We will not leave you. We will watch with you. We will be there.

4. Informational

Through great tribulation we have gained peace.

Anonymous

Informational support means providing patients, family members, other palliative caregivers and the general public information about palliative care, including how to provide physical, emotional, and spiritual support. This chapter is written for the caregivers who have constant opportunities to provide patients, families and non-palliative care providers with the information and skills they need to help someone who is dying.

Many people who are dying and their families crave information. Many want to know about their illness and how it will affect their lives until they die. Many want to know if they will suffer pain or intolerable symptoms. Many want some idea of how long they will live. Many want help in settling their estates, planning funerals, understanding how to work with the other members of the palliative care team and how to help each other (patient helping family and vice-versa).

People often crave this information at times when no one else is around. They want to understand what is happening to them when they are awake at three in the morning and everyone else is sleeping. Family members live in a society where their friends may not know how to provide practical support. All of these needs can be partly addressed by providing people with information.

There are many ways that this can, and should be done by all members of a palliative care team. The following are just some examples:

1. Have a 24-hour telephone number that people can call to get objective, up-to-date answers and support.
2. Have fact sheets that help patients and families and volunteers understand the probable development of specific diseases and the medications and treatment often used.
3. Have some case studies to describe in real terms how successful palliative care has been in similar circumstances being faced by the patient.
4. Have a lending library of books, videos, audio cassettes and articles that will help individuals who want more than basic information. This could include information on the truths and myths of dying and death, caregiver and patient-family stresses, how to provide day-to-day practical supports, how to plan funerals, and how to deal with financial and other legal matters.
5. Have a single sheet of paper or brochure with a list of the other professionals and volunteers on the team and how they can be reached.

6. Have time set aside on a regular basis (both professionals and volunteers) to answer the ongoing questions that patients and families will have. Help them remember your answers by providing written handouts that answer the more common, repetitive questions you get asked all the time. People only hear 20% of what you tell them and they forget 80% of that within a day so they have to have written reminders of important details. Encourage them to bring along another family member or friend when they meet with you. This person can take notes and help them remember important information.
7. Encourage those who are interested to get involved in other programs, service, or support groups. Such activities are not for most people who are dying or who are grieving the death of a loved one, but they do help some people.
8. Help teach families and friends the basics of practical nursing care for someone in the hospital and someone at home. Most often, patients who go home must rely on their family and friends who were probably asked to leave the hospital room when basic care was performed by nurses. Take all opportunities to teach those who want to learn about physical, emotional and spiritual care.

Information is like a safety net. It helps people understand what is happening to them, what is normal or abnormal about their reactions and condition and helps give them back some control over their lives which they may have lost during the earlier treatment of their illness.

Information gives people some predictability in their lives. While we are planning our lives months or even years in advance, people who are dying and their families are trying to get through the next few hours and days. They need some of the same predictability of the future that all of us need.

Information is often hoarded in health care. The assumption still exists that people are not capable of understanding or that there is too little time to communicate well. Palliative care was designed partly in response to that attitude. People must have the choice to know as much as they want about their illness, their future and their concerns. The patient and family must have access to information when they want it, versus when we want to give it to them (if at all).

Personal Comments 2

by Dorothy Ley

To Physicians

My professional background is that of a haematologist, oncologist and provider of palliative care. I believe it is important to make some direct comments to my colleagues from all medical disciplines.

Just because you have cared for a lot of people who have died does not make you an expert on dying or death. Physicians by nature are people who like to do everything themselves. That characteristic is reinforced by other experiences, including medical schools. I find it appalling that young physicians feel that they have failed when a patient dies. When we were granted our medical degrees we were not given the authority to give our patients eternal life, nor for that matter to take it away.

What then is palliative care from a physician's perspective? Palliative care is more than its simple definition. We learned (if we had any palliative care instruction at all) that to palliate means to relieve without curing; to medicate and to alleviate pain and symptoms to be best of our abilities. However, there is something wrong with the notion that presumes that a physician foregoes curative care when palliative care is instituted. We must recognize, I believe, that there are many physicians who assume that palliative care is really a concession to more mainline, vigorous cure-directed therapy. It is that attitude (which is fairly general and common) that has made it difficult to provide good care of people who are terminally ill.

Physicians must remember that death is one of only two events that all humans experience. At the same time it is a moment that each of us must experience alone. As Herman Feifel wrote, "To die is a human condition. To live decently and to die well is a privilege." Physicians often prevent people from dying well because of our training to cure first, care second. The palliative care philosophy encourages us to go back to the teachings of that great nineteenth century Canadian physician-teacher, Sir William Osler, who taught medical students that we must always treat both the mind and the body within each of our patients. In that way we allow people to live their lives in the way they chose before their death and, therefore, to have the privilege to die well.

Few physicians understand their role on a palliative care team. As a physician you have specialized knowledge and skills and so does every other team member. The major distinction is that physicians are usually legally responsible for a patient's care and, therefore, your role on a team cannot be equal to everyone else. Having said that, no physician has ever been charged with providing palliative care. On a practical, day-to-day level, you are equal to other members of the palliative care team and have an equal responsibility to learn the skills of team dynamics and how to help a team reach and maintain its full potential.

In palliative care, decisions rarely need to be made quickly. The patient, family and other caregivers that are part of the interdisciplinary team understand that the patient is dying and that care is primarily focused at comfort for the patient. Situations are more predictable in such a setting and decisions are made by consensus long before there are changes in the patient's condition. There are few unexpected emergency situations in palliative care and those that do happen can usually be handled without the need for group decision making because the team has already discussed similar situations in the past.

The danger happens when patients are referred to palliative care programs hours or days before their death and the team has not had time to develop a working relationship with the patient and family. Even in situations such as these, the compassion, team work and the team's experiences with such cases results in patients (when possible) and families feeling relieved that "the system" does indeed provide a compassionate, practical alternative to admission to emergency units or acute care treatments.

It is important to remember that no physician has ever been

convicted for providing palliative care in Canada. Although you are legally responsible for your patient, the interdisciplinary team approach reduces to a minimum any risks of providing palliative care in isolation.

Physicians, other health care providers and the public must lobby for changes in the physician fee structures for palliative care. In the mid-1980s it was estimated that a family physician caring for terminally ill people and billing the Ontario Hospital Insurance Plan under its schedule at the time would have difficulty making $25,000 a year if he or she worked seven days per week without any holidays. It has not changed substantially enough since then. Until, and unless, major reforms are made in the method of payment for physician services across Canada the development of palliative care will be severely, and damagingly, restricted.

To All Professional Caregivers

My background is medical so I will not give specific comments to professionals from other disciplines. However, there are a few specific things that I think are important to say to all caregivers who provide palliative care including some comments on the ethics of care.

It is very difficult to put together an interdisciplinary team. Not a team that is just a collection of people with different disciplinary backgrounds. You must each learn the skills of team dynamics and commit yourself to actively participating in that team dynamic to increase communication, to share responsibility and to resolve conflicts as they arise.

As with physicians, you need to constantly enhance your professional skills, especially as they apply to palliative patients. The knowledge and skills within palliative care are increasing worldwide as new ideas, techniques and procedures are developed. Our patients and their families count on us to be up-to-date on ways to help them through their final life's journey.

Everyone on the team must understand their own strengths and weaknesses. You can never do everything equally well for a patient and their family. Therefore, learn to ask for help in areas where you are least comfortable and teach others your areas of strength. There are no rules that say physicians must always give "bad news" or that spiritual leaders are the only ones who can talk about God and an afterlife. If you feel yourself holding back your expertise, make an extra effort to share your knowledge and skills.

Palliative care providers have an extra onus to examine their own beliefs about dying, death, spirituality, the meaning of life and dealing with grief. You cannot take emotional and spiritual suffering away from someone but you can understand, somewhat, what others are feeling and help them to help themselves. Understand how your spiritual beliefs may help, or hinder, a patient's own beliefs. Never preach your own beliefs but use those beliefs to help join a common bond of spirituality with the patient, if they chose to have you involved in that way.

Never lose sight of the palliative care philosophy of care: provide the physical, emotional, spiritual and informational supports that patients and families need, when they need them. There will be times when it will be more comforting, or easy, to concentrate on writing reports, presenting policy papers to government or other funders, in doing public education, debating doctor-assisted suicide, etc. Constantly ask yourself: "Who am I doing this for? How will this directly affect the people I know who are dying now? While I am doing this, who is caring for people who are dying?"

A last thought – the demands on palliative care will increase in the next few decades. You may be involved in helping more and more people. Your annual reports will be filled with impressive statistics of how many people you helped that year. Remind yourself that the hospice movement in Canada began in response to health care systems that forgot how to care for people who were dying. If you cannot remember the names of the patients you are serving, perhaps you are serving too many. Perhaps we will need to concentrate on helping people within the community return to a time (not that long ago) when caring for people who were dying was a privilege and part of the seasonal lives of people in a community. Rather than build empires or be funded by health care empires, perhaps, we need to remember people like Bill, Sue, Nasreen, Geovanni, Michelle and Juan Carlos – the people who rely on us at one of the most vulnerable times in their lives. We have made dramatic differences in the lives of individuals in Canada because we got to know them as people.

To Volunteers

Volunteers can do so many things. The fact that you are not paid means that your involvement is a true, freely-given gift. You need to understand the philosophy of hospice care and how you can best fulfil it with your own unique sets of knowledge, interests and skills. The important role that volunteers can play is that you are able to meet the needs of patients, as defined by the individual patient and advocate on their behalf when necessary. You have no professional affiliation nor are you a paid staff of a particular service, therefore, you can afford to be loyal to the person who is ill rather than primarily loyal to the service where you volunteer.

The relationship between professional caregivers and volunteers is not well defined. On the one hand, some families and professional caregivers treat volunteers as professionals and, on the other hand, they treat them as unimportant. The volunteer, in a way, is the cement that holds the palliative care service together. He or she brings part of the patient's world to the team that professionals cannot do. No matter how hard professionals try, they must play the roles expected of them by the patient, their profession and other professionals. The volunteer has no such inhibitions.

But we must beware. We must beware not to use them to fill up the economic chinks and pick up the funding pieces, as it were. We must beware that we develop and apply appropriate ways of choosing volunteers for the setting in which they are going to work. That setting may be an institution or it may be a home. We must carefully examine the role of the volunteer in those various settings and the way that role various from one to another. We must develop training programs that are appropriate to the settings. In fact, much of this work has started in Canada but we must be vigilant in ensuring long-term accountability of all members of the palliative care team, including volunteers. We must be certain that we know the legal and ethical implications of the volunteer's activities in palliative care. We must above all support them, train them, and be certain that, wherever they work, they are full, integrated members of the team.

The second way in which voluntarism is important in palliative care is in funding. There is a grass roots movement in this country to take palliative care out of the institutions and into the community. It has taken the form of the development of volunteer, community based hospice programs. Some of these programs or services are designed to help patients in their homes while others help patients in hospitals or free-standing hospices (such as Casey House in Toronto). Some of these services include the services of professionals within the service while others work along side professionals in the community.

I happen to believe personally that public involvement in the delivery of care, particularly in an area like palliative care, is a good thing. I keep going back to the philosophy of palliative care. If we really believe that we can only deliver palliative care in terms of a person who lives within a family and a community then we cannot trap that care in an institution. It has to get out into the community somehow. Palliative care units in some hospitals will be necessary to provide special pain and symptom control, respite care and a safe environment for people who cannot stay at home. These units are also necessary to help teach other caregivers the specifics of palliative care that can not be taught in the community as easily.

People are becoming increasingly disenchanted, however, with the way in which the elderly are cared for, the chronically ill are housed, and the terminally ill treated. There is an increasing need to be involved in the care of these people. But that need should be channelled. We should be planning for the development of mixed volunteer and professional groups out in communities. We should be examining the reasoning for the apparent need (or lack of it) for alternatives such as free-standing hospices, especially in rural communities where modern health care is too far away from home.

Right now across Canada there is a growing number of free-standing hospices being planned. Property and buildings have been purchased. Who knows how inappropriate these may be? The response of governments will be to deny them access to funds and in some situations to deny them the right to operate. I am not at all sure that hospices are the right way to go. However, I think all of us who work in the field of palliative care should be examining the options and helping to make plans for the future that meet the needs of individuals who are dying within their own communities. There are no generic answers that fit all communities and all needs. We can not possibly depend on volunteer money for operating a program. However, there must be a place for it within that system.

Co-operation is essential if we are to develop an integrated system of palliative care in this country. I also believe that future planning will have to focus on community- based services whenever possible. Institutional programs may remain necessary for training and research purposes and for exceptional situations where a person cannot, or chooses not to, stay at home. These programs may include free-standing hospices and palliative care units within hospitals.

On the Ethics of Care

There are some fundamental ethical issues that are associated with the practice of palliative care that we ignore at our peril. Perhaps the discipline of palliative care can take the lead in helping society solve some of these problems.

We are caught between the philosophy of "triage" – husband scarce resources and use them only where they will do the most good – and the Hippocratic Oath – care for all who need your care, regardless of cost. We say, "I am my brother's keeper" while grim economic reality says, "We can't take care of everyone equally – make a choice". One of the very real tensions in palliative care today is just that: How do we make a choice without compromising our philosophy of care, or our ethics. Or can we?

Whether we like it or not, when combined with rapidly changing demographics, the economic constraints in our society are forcing us to face the dilemma of age-related access to care. Is palliative care going to be available only for the young when 70% of people in palliative care are over the age of 65? Will it be limited to people who share similar views on health, illness and death as the leaders within the palliative care movement? Who makes these decisions and on what grounds? Do those ethical grounds reflect the beliefs and values of Canadians or of the medical and bioethical communities?

There are others more qualified than I to discuss the difficult ethical problems of "do not resuscitate orders" (DNR) and euthanasia. Let me remind you, however, that the increasing demand for legalized living wills and for euthanasia is a reflection of the fact that the public trusts neither the caregivers nor the system.

The phrase "dying with dignity" means different things to different people. For some it means dying with their own clothes on and in full possession of their faculties. For others, it is the absence of pain and difficult symptoms. For others, it is the end to a life lived with dignity. The current fashion to equate dying with dignity with euthanasia reflects the mistaken belief that death whose moment is chosen is somehow more dignified that one not chosen.

We must remember that death is rarely dignified as we have come to define dignity. People's bodies change and begin to lose control over normal functions. This was once seen as a natural process and not one to avoid, isolate or terminate. Dignity is also an inherent quality that can not be given to someone else and certainly not at the end of their lives. Dignity can be taken away from people, however, by taking away their right to make decisions, to prevent them from taking part in their own palliative care and by converting the concept of "the right to die" with a "duty to die."

People at the margins of life – those who are poor, elderly, illiterate, immigrants, of non- Christian faiths, women, of colour, with disabilities – are already at great risk of dying. The duty to die is increased with economic constraints on health care. Legalized euthanasia or medically-assisted suicide would make that duty all the more pervasive, regardless of all the supposed safeguards mentioned by others. If you think this is not true, remember that hospitals and health care systems embody the attitudes of society. In our death-denying western hospitals, cure is still more important than care. Our professional training, our allocation of resources and our attitudes towards, and the treatment of, the terminally ill, the incurable and the elderly are predicated on the importance of cure. We isolate the dying and reject and institutionalize the elderly.

The demand for euthanasia is a desperate response to an intolerable situation. Change the response or the situation and the demands fade. I firmly believe that it is the role of hospice or palliative care to represent that change in response and to alter the situation. Palliative care is not a response to euthanasia. Both palliative care and euthanasia are responses to health care systems that do not meet the needs of people who are dying. Once we understand that distinction perhaps society and its media will understand the purpose and practical supports that the palliative care philosophy offers us all.

One last comment: the debate over euthanasia, to me, is an

example of the lack of thoughtfulness and perception of the difference between killing yourself or someone else and providing a dignified, peaceful death. They are quite different. I think it is a disgrace that someone can flog an unprofessional book on how to kill yourself and make a million dollars on it. I think it is a sad comment on our society when we will spend millions of dollars buying books that help us to kill ourselves, or others, and only thousands of dollars to help provide compassionate palliative care. The public demand at present is for doctor-assisted suicide or euthanasia because they do not understand that dying with dignity comes through dying without pain, alert and with your emotional and spiritual needs supported by people who will walk the journey with you. Our politicians, to date, follow the opinion polls and, therefore, have not provided the leadership we need to educate all Canadians about the real choices available to us. Nor have political leaders, and other leaders in this drive toward legalizing euthanasia done systematic, empirical studies to examine the probable consequences of euthanasia legislation. We may spend millions of dollars a year on environmental studies to safeguard nature (as we should) but no one is suggesting we spend some dollars to safeguard humanity as well. A tragic situation.

Conclusions

I have built a wall of laughter
Around the house of my heart.
Grow old along with me.
The best is yet to be.
The last of life for which the first was made:
Our times are in His hand.

Robert Browning

As each of us comes to the end of our life – whether it was a short life or a long one – we must pass through the door that leads from this life to a life beyond. That door is death. Not one of us approaches it alone. We are accompanied by our loves, our hates, our ambitions, our fears, our faith (or lack of it), by our successes and our failures. We are accompanied by all the memories, the myriad of people, places and events that have shaped our lives.

It is not an easy approach for anyone. No matter how firm our faith, how strong our support, not one of us can help but look back at all we have known with longing and look forward with some apprehension – and sometimes with fear.

What is palliative care? It is the paving of that final road – whether it be made up of small bright pieces or large solid stones. The mosaic of palliative care provides the support and marks the way for all those for whom we care. You are the cement – you are the glue that holds it together. All of you who are part of the delivery of hospice or palliative care, whether you be professionals, volunteers, community or family members. Diverse, multi-faceted, inter-mingled – you are as different and as unique as the many parts of the mosaic. It is your love, your caring, your commitment, your skills and knowledge that hold the pieces together and make them strong.

Hospice care stands as a model for tolerance at the final moment of truth in everyone's life. The challenge to hospice in the years ahead is to take a deeply religious, fervently Christian (Judeo-Christian), uniquely Anglo-Saxon philosophy of care and apply it successfully to radically different situations. This will require discipline, compassion and understanding, vision, and above all, faith.

My philosophic approach to patients throughout my practice was the palliative care philosophy. It was taught to me by good men and women clinicians who cared about their patients. It was not restricted to patients who were dying but for all patients. The fact that now it is restricted to people who have a terminal illness is appalling. We should be teaching the philosophy of hospice care in public school and in society and, of course, in health care sciences. It should be taught – period.

The challenge to hospice is to reach out to each other and strengthen and support each others' roles on that much vaunted inter-disciplinary team – not to compete with the belief that one's own profession is somehow better able to meet the needs of people who are dying. We all have personal and professional strengths and none of us, regardless of our background, can provide palliative care on our own.

The challenge is to reach out to people who need palliative care in parts of this country that are hard and difficult and where there is little monetary return – in the far north and in the slums of our cities. We must reach out to the communities beyond the borders of those cities, to the small towns, to the countryside, where there are people who want to die in their own homes surrounded by family and friends but where there is almost no professional help and no money to provide it.

We need to reach out to the marginalized in our society – to the elderly, to people with AIDS, to recognize and to meet their needs.

Finally, the challenge to hospice is to recognize the spirituality in each of us, no matter what our religion, to share in it and to work to make your own spirituality grow and deepen by the exchange.

The mosaic of palliative care, dark pieces and bright pieces, uneven in shape, irregular in design all become part of a pattern – a pattern of care. You will decide by what you do and how you do it whether it will become a mosaic that will ultimately include all health and social care. The choice is yours.

Remember, in hospice's search for scientific excellence, the creation of standards, the demands for formalized education and government funding for care, (all appropriate and necessary), we must never forget to reach out beyond ourselves, beyond our personal pride and ambition, beyond our turf, if you like, to reach out from our inner self to the people for whom we care – all of them. For love, is the litmus test of palliative care and spirituality is its heart. "Love," wrote Buckminster Fuller, "is omni-inclusive, progressively exquisite, understanding and tender, and compassionately attuned to other than self."

Part II

Hospice Success Stories

Hospice Care Success Stories 3

by Harry van Bommel

This chapter includes success stories in palliative care from across Canada. We begin with Dr. Dorothy Ley's own success story of how she lived her life as she wanted until her death January 31, 1994. The rest of the stories in this chapter are a testament to some of the impact that Dorothy Ley had on the how people receive care in the last months of their lives.

Dorothy Ley's own experience with cancer began in 1983 and became more serious in 1990. For the last three years of her life she went through numerous treatments including surgery, radiation and chemotherapy – some of it experimental. Throughout this time she chaired a major review of palliative care in Metropolitan Toronto for the District Health Council, continued to sit on various committees, write articles and give speeches, and influence the course of events in Canadian Palliative Care and care of our elders.

By the Fall of 1993, it became clear that further treatment would be more harmful than helpful. She remained under the care of her oncologist and the palliative care team at Oshawa General Hospital. Together they managed her pain and symptoms and gave her the freedom to fulfil a few dreams she still had.

One such dream was to travel to her nephew's wedding in Calgary by first flying to Vancouver and taking the train through the Rocky Mountains. She had once travelled through the Rockies at night and had promised to one day see them by train during the day. Her courage and determination to complete this trip alone still astound some of her closest friends.

Another dream had been to have one more Christmas as she had traditionally celebrated this high holiday in the past. As always, she went to have Christmas Eve dinner with her friends the Oldenziel family. The family had offered to go to Dorothy's home to make it easier for her but she refused. She enjoyed her evening with the family and the evening service at church. On Christmas day she remained alone for the most of the day as she wanted. Many friends called to wish her well and she spent the remainder of the day enjoying the beauty of her beloved home and the beautiful nature all around it. With this dream fulfilled she left the next day for Oshawa General Hospital where her illness quickly overtook her. She had been determined to be at home as long as possible but knew when it was time to get the extra help she needed during the last month of her life.

During her care she always asked to be treated as a patient; not a doctor. She wanted care, comfort and support rather than collegial rapport. With other patients she always served the role as helpful doctor so that they might receive even better service, but for herself she asked to be treated as Dorothy Ley, not Dr. Ley.

The palliative care team at the hospital became a second family to Dorothy. They usually prepare a room for a patient when they know they are coming in. They would have a lazy boy chair for comfort, a special mattress for the bed, a radio, fresh flowers, etc. When Dorothy was leaving after one of her monthly chemotherapy visits, the team asked her if there was anything else she would like waiting for her on her next visit. She replied that balloons would be nice and then laughed. Sure enough, on her next visit there was a bouquet of balloons in her room with pictures of butterflies (the team's logo) and flowers on the balloons. Everyone enjoyed the friendliness that such efforts bring out in people.

Dorothy's pain and symptoms were well controlled even though Dorothy took only tiny amounts of pain medication. Later in her illness she would become drowsy but that was a result of her cancer, especially the cancer in her liver, rather than from her medication.

During her last month in the hospital, Dorothy's condition was very serious and her friends and the palliative care team were not sure if she would be able to go home as she had wished. However, she rallied and was able to go home on Tuesday, January 25th. The palliative care team were very sad to see her leave as they had become very close to her and would not be close enough to provide her home support. They knew, of course, that Dorothy had always expressed a desire to be at home at the end of her life and they were very pleased that they were able to make the wish come true.

Dorothy had not planned who would take care of her at home when she would be unable to care for herself. Those who knew and loved her just naturally became more and more involved as they were needed. They were supported by St. Elizabeth Visiting Nurses who provided whatever nursing care was required. Many more people offered to help than was practical to accommodate but it showed how many people really cared for Dorothy.

Dorothy knew that she was going home and thoroughly enjoyed being in the place filled with so many happy memories. Her dog Sheena was able to visit several times and a friend hung up a bird feeder outside her bedroom window. For the first few days at home she was able to enjoy the company of people around her. She became progressively weaker but was comfortable throughout that last week at home. She enjoyed music playing throughout the day and night and particularly enjoyed Handel's Water Music, Mozart, "Solitudes" music mixed with nature sounds, and other quiet reflective music.

Dorothy was constantly surrounded by a few close friends. She had asked that they "just be there" with her, and they were. On Monday, January 31st she became increasingly quiet. She had been semi-conscious for the last few days but now her breathing was becoming more peaceful and quiet. There were no rattling sounds, no disquieting movements, and within a short time she died in comfort and peace as the sun was setting outside her window.

Dorothy once wrote that she "expected to get care that will relieve suffering whether that suffering be physical, emotional or spiritual. It is out there for me. It is allowing me the privilege and support I need to make my own decisions about my life until I die and to come to terms with my own death." Her family, friends and palliative care providers fulfilled her expectations with love, skill and understanding.

* * *

The following stories are quoted from works done by participants at a workshop on promoting palliative care more actively. This workshop was held at the Canadian Palliative Care Conference in Winnipeg, Manitoba in the Fall of 1993. The writers have given their permission to allow anyone in the field of palliative care to reproduce these stories to promote palliative care. The names of people in some of the stories have been changed to protect their privacy and some writers asked that their own name not be acknowledged, again to protect the privacy of the people presented. You do not need to ask for permission to use this copyrighted material. We do ask that you acknowledge the writer's name of each specific story and acknowledge that you found the story in this book. I am grateful to the writers who allow all of us to share in their success stories.

"Jack"

by Judy Galenza

When Jack was diagnosed with pancreatic cancer, he seemed to know his prognosis immediately. He was 43 years old, with two small boys and a wife. He knew their time together was going to be limited. Unlike most others with a terminal illness, Jack did not pursue "wonder cures." He told his doctor he would see him later because he had some living left to do.

The next few months, Jack continued to be an active member of his family. He continued to accept responsibility for his own health and learned to operate intravenous and pain medication infusion pumps. Frequently, you would see Jack inspect and drain his stomach tube and report back to medical personnel on its function. He seemed to feel if he had control of the bulk of his care, he could still assume control in other areas of his life – those areas being a father to his children and a husband to his wife.

Despite a growing physical weakness, Jack had a determination to be present at his boys' soccer games and to cheer them from the sidelines. Together with his wife's assistance, they managed to infuse his intravenous fluids as quickly and as early in the day as possible so he could continue sharing time with his family. The advancement in pain management also kept him comfortable throughout the day so he was able, and felt like being, an active player in his family.

As the cancer in Jack's body grew, his roles and responsibilities to his family lessened. Jack made a choice early in his diagnosis to stay at home and be cared for with the help of his wife, physician and Home Care. I am pleased to say that Jack's wish was fulfilled and he died peacefully in the comfort of his own home and in the presence of his family. Everyone involved in this story considers Jack a success and he is a reminder to all of us that "dying is not an illness, it is a process."

"Mom"

by Shirley Kloon

Caregiving has traditionally and historically been a role assumed by women. We've had the natural aspirations of nurturing. My story is about my three brothers who provided compassionate and creative care to our mother who was dying.

I, being the only daughter, knew that I would not be able to provide all the care. Two of my brothers were married but when I approached them about caring for our mother, I told them that if they agreed to my proposal/suggestion, they could not pass this task on to their wives. We developed a schedule so everyone would be able to be with Mom at home at a time that it would be best for each of us. In order to give them a sense of security, I volunteered to be available at all times. Since I was a nurse, I was supposed to be an expert – the one who would know what to do if they needed help.

I am sorry that I didn't involve my brothers sooner. They were creative, innovative and fun. Our mother enjoyed being cared for by her family at her home. Her own mother, siblings and friends and neighbours were able to come and go at leisure. There were no visiting hours and if she needed to rest we just recessed to the kitchen and living room. When she awoke she would call for us to return or she would listen to the conversation from her room.

One day, one of my brothers set up a temporary bed by the large dining room window and moved Mom to this area to enjoy the sunshine and view of the yard. When the priest came to visit her, he went to the room where Mom had her bed. He was shocked to see it empty and thought she had died. My brother called him to the dining room where he soon realized that she indeed was still alive and alert. This small joke on Father Frank particularly amused our mother and, indeed, raised her spirits.

Their cooking and cleaning generally needed Mom's assistance and advice on how to do this or that around her home in her way. It was very heart warming for her to have her sons care this much about how she preferred things done. She was able to maintain control of her home rather than having some "other woman" coming in and taking over.

I learned that we need to involve the males in our families in caregiving. Given the chance, they can express their love and care in ways that no woman can.

"Mark"

by Alex Heuser

Mark was a man in his early 70s. He was a construction worker. He had lost his wife to cancer a few years ago and he was now dying himself due to cancer. He was being cared for in a hospital palliative care unit and it was during this time that I, as a volunteer, came to know him.

During our first visit, Mark told me quite a lot about his life, including both highlights and disappointments. Most strikingly of all, he told me that he had "one month left." As well, he was quite interested in that fact that I am a blind person and felt comfortable asking questions regarding how I manage life's tasks. I answered his questions and in so doing attempted to dispel any possible thought that I was super smart or brave. Instead, I shared my belief that each one of us seems to find the courage and strength to do what we have to do. I explained that I visit the unit every Tuesday and Mark asked to see me again the next week.

During our second and third visits, Mark continued to share his life with me including: the onset of his illness; the hope and despair felt with each unsuccessful medical attempt to curb the illness; and his appreciation for the nursing care which has kept him physically comfortable. Of his five children, he talked most about Ron (age 21 – youngest of the family) with whom he had been living and to whom he had already given all of his limited possessions.

Our third visit was highlighted by Mark's excitement over Ron having become engaged the previous evening and also because Ron had come to visit that same evening and brought his fiancee to meet him. Mark's feeling of joy, even relief, in now knowing that all his children had a partner was abundantly obvious.

During our fourth visit and following a bit of casual talk, Mark asked if I would like some fish. My inner sense told me that maybe Mark was wanting to give me some fish but I couldn't imagine from where unless it was left over from lunch. Not being too fond of fish, I wanted to decline the offer, but somehow I knew to accept. I had no sooner replied when Mark leaped from his bed, went to the family room/kitchen and returned with a plate of food and a glass of juice for me. The food consisted of some green salad, a slice of buttered bread and a cold but cooked fillet of pickerel. The food was delicious and as I ate Mark told me stories from some of his fishing trips. The meal eaten and my appreciation appropriately expressed, Mark then explained that an out-of-town cousin had brought the home-prepared food to him.

This visit being the fourth one, I recalled with Mark that when we first met he had told me that he had a month left. I told him that I surely hoped to see him next week but, just in case, we could say our "good-bye" now – which we did. Mark died six days later. From Mark I learned two very basic things: (1) listen to the inner sense – it is usually correct; and (2) be aware of how wonderful it must feel to do something for someone else when one has become so dependant on others because of illness. I will always be thankful for the opportunity of having been Mark's last lunch guest.

"The Death of My Father"

by Claire (Burris) Noseworthy

My father, at age 86, was dying from that commonly dreaded disease, cancer. Although he spoke no words, his wish was to be cared for at home. We understood his silent plea because he had completely irrational behaviour every time he entered the hospital, but had a warm satisfied expression of peace when he was back at home.

My father was a General Practitioner who started his medical practice when most of medicine centred around home care. He was lucky enough to be the first doctor liaison in starting up the official home care program in our small community. Our family was lucky to have two nurses amongst the four of us; my mother making three. So it was with the help of home care, a dedicated friend who was a physician, and the mutual support of the remaining family that we were able to keep Father at home and let him die in peace.

For approximately three months, off and on, he required complete bed care. It was a privilege for me to be able to do this for him. My brother, when visiting one day, suggested perhaps Dad would feel more at ease if we let the home care nurse give him his bed bath and his response was, "Oh no, I much prefer my own nurses." It was easy for all of us and I now treasure those moments of touching and caring.

Dying was easy for him. He had a wonderful outlook on both life and death. He once said to me, "Dear, there are only two guarantees in life. You are born and you will die. We don't have a lot of control over either so make the most out of the time in between. God doesn't bring you into this world with a guarantee of 65 years of healthy fun. It's up to you to make the most of each day." So he was ready at 86 to die – he had no regrets. He stated calmly one day, "I'm ready. I feel I have fulfilled all my reasonable obligations."

Although dying was easy, the process of getting there, however, was not. He once said, "Dying is not formidable, but this pain is unbearable." At first it was a major challenge to convince him to take any medication but quite honestly I think he was grateful to finally let us give him injections at regular intervals. He was a stoic and resisted, vehemently, taking anything himself.

We celebrated when he finally ceased breathing and I swear the undertaker has never recovered from the likes of the Burris family!

To live is to die. My father's living and his dying were an inspiration to many.

"Morgan"

by Patricia Collins

I couldn't wait to get the results of my pregnancy test. In my heart,

I knew it was positive but I waited patiently for the report before I spread the good news. The pregnancy was quite uneventful except for the feeling of nausea that accompanied each day. My husband and I visited the doctor each month. I watched my diet and tried to live as healthy as possible.

Toward the end of the pregnancy, we took Lamaze classes to prepare us for our due date. That date arrived and so did a healthy 7 pound 2 ounce boy. We were quite pleased since there were no complications and everything went as it should have. That is until the day before we were to go home. The doctor detected a heart murmur and because the hospital did not have the equipment to do an echocardiogram, we were flown 500 miles to a facility that could do the test. That day is very blurry. I couldn't understand how this could be happening but even though I was scared, I was hopeful.

Very shortly after our arrival, the test was done and I was told that this healthy-looking baby boy was not going to live. I remember very little after that. I was numb. I guess I was in shock. He was placed in the neonatal unit and we were given a small room on the same floor. We didn't know what to do. We had so many questions that no one could answer. Why? How long? How was it going to be at the end? Can we take him home? He had a hypoplastic left heart which meant that vital parts of his heart were not developed and eventually his heart would stop working.

The medical and nursing staff were kind and compassionate but did not understand what we were going through. It was left up to us. It was very difficult but we decided to go home if the hospital there would re-admit Morgan. This was arranged and also I was going to be able to stay on a medical ward in the hospital that was closed so I could be near to breast feed. When we arrived at the hospital, Morgan was readmitted but no arrangements had been made for me. We ended up staying at a motel nearby to be awakened when Morgan awoke to be breast fed.

We were exhausted, confused and most of all, we were angry. We were going through this terrible experience and it seemed that we had to work harder to make decisions because of the lack of support.

I think it was partly the anger we felt that helped us make the decision to take Morgan home. Even though that decision was made out of anger and confusion, it was the best decision we ever made. We took him home and everything changed. We were able to take care of him and establish a routine for the three of us – we were a real family. Friends and neighbours and, in particular, family were able to come and meet Morgan and visit. Morgan lived for nine days and died a peaceful death in the arms of his Mom and Dad.

"Never Lose Your Smile"

by Kim Kerr

Ann was a very special person. She is someone who walked into my life, touched it and kept leaving a huge gift behind.

Ann was diagnosed with a re-occurrence of cancer. She was told her condition was terminal and that, unlike the last time, there was nothing they could do to stop the cancer cells. Ann was angry. She felt betrayed by the medical system who only a few years earlier told her she had a clean bill of health. Ann shared this anger towards all who cared for her and her family.

Ann's family was persistent that they could, and would, care for her at home. They wanted to give back all they had shared and be a part of her death. Ann wanted no part of this for her family. She packed her small tweed suitcase and told all involved she was going to the hospital to stay and die. Her family became very frustrated but agreed with her wishes. They visited frequently but they were angry and discouraged.

Ann was diagnosed by her caregivers as having "Ringitis." She rang her call bell frequently and demanded to have her needs met. Staff became very discouraged and nurses were shocked. All available resources were utilized. Debriefing sessions were held regularly with staff. Brainstorming was done with regards to providing the best care possible. Palliative care conferences between physicians, social worker, clergy and staff were held regularly but all involvement in care was discouraged and "sent away" by Ann.

Nothing seemed to improve. Ann became more demanding and bitter towards us and nothing seemed to be resolvable with her family.

The part I played in Ann's care was as a staff nurse. I had become frustrated with her care. I tried on numerous occasions to "open the door" for communication and time and time again was unsuccessful.

One evening as we heard the buzzer ring for the twentieth time, I said to a co-worker, "It's okay. It's my turn to walk on pins and needles." I took a deep breath and put a smile on my face. I walked into her room. She yelled at me to do some menial tasks and said, "And, take that fake smile off your face." Under my breath I laughed and to my amazement, she laughed too. I turned around quickly to make sure it was a laugh and not a hiccup and to my amazement she was laughing. We both laughed together.

She said to me, "Of all the nurses, I can tell that you have a lot of people who love you." I put down her side rail and sat with her (I took her hand) and we talked. We talked about her anger, her feelings at losing control and how she felt her family let her down by not understanding and by doing what they thought was right versus what she thought was right. We closed our conversation with her saying, "I have decided to let you care for me. Remember all those that love you and show them love. Whatever you do, do not lose your smile."

Ann's journey towards death had taught me so much. Her constant struggle for control in a setting where so much was taken away was so evident. Once Ann decided to let us help her die and once we realized that she was the leader, our care was well received. Her memory will be with me always. Her death was peaceful, surrounded by family and friends.

"Mr. C."

by John Mowry

Upon returning from vacation this past May I learned of a 40-year-old man who had been referred to our program. Mr. C. lived with his wife and three daughters in a small agricultural community; the prime reference point in town was the flashing amber light on the main street.

I first met the family in their home in my role as a social worker who sees patients both in their homes and in the hospital. The home was modest but comfortable. I quickly learned that what was important to the family was their relationship to one another and their attachment to their land and their horses. The home was surrounded by mountains of sage, wild flowers and riding trails.

I asked what was different for the children since their father had become sick. The oldest (10 years old) told me of how she couldn't go horseback riding with her father anymore. The middle daughter (7 years old) spoke about her father who took care of her when her mom was sick and wondered who would care for them if she became sick again since her dad was too sick to help. The youngest daughter (2 1/2) sat on her father's lap. All the children lamented that they had extra chores to do!

As the weeks passed, Mr. C. became increasingly ill. The children wanted factual information about their father's cancer. What colour, size and shape was it? What operation did he have? I was able to share specific information obtained from the hospital's pathologist. On one of my visits I commented on the horse pendant that the oldest daughter was wearing. She told me it was given to her from a classmate at school. She had written a story describing what it was like for her, watching and caring for her father who was dying of cancer. She said one of the boys started to cry as she read her story. A few days later he gave her the necklace she was wearing in hopes of making her feel better. Mr. C. died at home, quietly, in his own bed. His two oldest daughters had been sitting with him, on the bed, just hours before he died. Extended family were present and I had been there earlier in the day.

Mr. C.'s brother had built a coffin. Mrs. C. phoned me to say her husband had died through the night. The girls were picking sage and wild flowers to put into the coffin which was in the family's front room. By the afternoon, the coffin was removed from the home and taken to the crematorium.

Follow-up meetings with the family leave me with an optimism and faith that relationships are enduring, if ever changing. They are working hard to discover and define their "new family." The two oldest girls continue to write about what they have experienced and are experiencing. Their mother is searching for her identity as a single parent. It will be through their searching, writing and sharing with others that they will make this family true ambassadors of Palliative Care.

"Helen"

Anonymous

Helen was a 64-year-old "bag" lady. The doctor and I walked her from an emergency shelter to our small six-bed hospice three blocks away. Helen's pain from cancer of the urethra was severe. Her world was one of paranoid schizophrenia and the streets. Her anguish was that the "inhumans" were burning her insides. Her pain distraction, for it can hardly be called management, was to create a topical pain consisting of brushing her perineum with no less than a hair brush.

For three days she sat curled, still in outdoor clothes, in a chair with her leg bent under her while she talked of the cruel inhumans that had taken her over. She refused to even look at any pills being offered that would help get rid of her inhumans.

On day three the break came, to our astonishment. Helen made no fuss or refusal when liquid medications were offered. Another 24 hours brought pain relief and, within a week after, antipsychotics had also been added to her regime. We had the most beautiful, friendly lady as part of our family.

Now Helen was still a little confused as to the number of children she had. "I know I had two," she said, "but you never know what happens at night so perhaps I have four." Helen's sister, who we had managed to track down, would have nothing to do with her and certainly was not about to give us any information. So for many weeks we kept asking Helen questions that might give us some more concrete information about her children. Another break came. Her sister actually called us and became more cooperative. During the next week we managed to track down one of Helen's children, her daughter, living in Saskatchewan. conversations were stilted at first. Donna had been searching for her mother for almost 15 years and was quite overwhelmed to find her but also overwhelmed that she was terminally ill with so little time to live.

Donna had a husband and children and she wanted desperately to see her mother. The family was living on welfare and could not afford the trip. A few weeks before, our hospice had received a donation from a grateful family. We decided that no better use could be made of the money than to pay for Donna and her family to drive out and spend a few days with us in our province.

The reunion was dramatically simple and beautiful and during the three days they were together a bond was reborn and many pictures were taken. Helen died three weeks later, sadly, very shortly before her 65th birthday. Her pension cheque, she told us, was going to make her a rich woman and she was going to share it with us and Donna.

Two years later we still hear from Donna. Her letters are full of love, and now understanding of why her mother had abandoned her all those years ago when she was thirteen. How much more fulfilled could we be too!

"Mary"

by Patricia Bray

Coping with short-term cancer can sometimes be catastrophic from the view of the few days you have to prepare the client and the family. Coping with long-term cancer (4-5 years) can be just as catastrophic since the client has prepared for death, it did not come, and now what do you do?

Mary had cancer and was on oral chemotherapy for a few years. During this time she did a lot of repairs and renovations to her home to have everything ready for her family when she died.

Mary developed a new tumour site in the lung and had it surgically removed and returned home. She felt she had battled cancer several times and this was just one more crisis. By this time, her family was completely exhausted. The family physician had not referred Mary to the palliative care program because she had come through so many crises before. He felt she would probably make it through this one too.

The daughter had given up work to look after her mother. She called me when she was at the "breaking point." After an hour's discussion on how the program could benefit her and her mother she decided to ask the doctor to refer her mother.

Mary was a very private person so we entered her life and her home very slowly and gently. When all the support systems were in place, a family conference was held and open discussion showed other members of the family how they could help the mother and daughter.

Mary remained at home, had several major crises in her last month of living, and the necessary services came to her home to help her. Her only real fear was going to the hospital. The daughter was very competent and functioned much better now that she had help.

Mary died peacefully at home with her family around her. A few days after her death, the daughter was asked by the physician what she thought of palliative care. She replied that she couldn't understand why she had not been referred to the program long ago. Maybe she wouldn't have had to quit her job. Maybe she could have had more patience with her mother had she not been so worn down from coping with the situation for such a long time by herself. In the grief recovery period, the daughter felt very much at peace that her mother had her wish to remain at home throughout her illness and death.

"Christmas in September"

Anonymous

Sarah lived (perhaps still lives) on the banks of the winding river with a Micmac name which means "Abundance" or "Paradise" depending on whom one asks. She was 78 and she was dying. She had raised nine children, all of whom cherished their mother; none of whom wanted her to know she was dying. All caregivers were warned not to tell her. A family member always sat outside the bedroom door in case one of us thought we would tell Sarah of her illness.

One day Sarah asked to see the Hospice Coordinator ALONE. She ordered everyone outside her room and outside of the house.

"Am I dying?"

"What do you think?"

"I think I am."

"Do you want to discuss what you think with your doctor or your family?"

"Answer me honestly. Will I live until Christmas, in your opinion?"

"No."

"Thank you very much! I love Christmas and I must hurry to

celebrate it one more time. They (my family) need never know you've told me."

Following our conversation, Sarah set about preparing for Christmas. She wrapped, with volunteer help, collections of spoons, thimbles, salt and pepper shakers, coins, and various other precious, personal items in bright yuletide paper. Appropriate name tags were added; a Christmas tree was cut and decorated; a marvellous holiday dinner was prepared and everyone was invited.

One daughter on the other side of Canada sent a tape of Christmas greetings to which the other children added their memories of Christmases past. The tape was placed under the tree for their mother.

Sarah celebrated Christmas on September 2nd with food, songs and gifts among those she loved most. Sarah died peacefully and with gentle acceptance on September 4, knowing she had given another Christmas full of memories to her family and had been able to divide her personal belongings among them as she wished – a living will. She had often remarked that although she and her husband had had the opportunity to travel extensively, she had always been happy to return home and sit in her sun porch overlooking the River of Abundance. She would say, "I am content to live and die in this beautiful land which truly is Paradise to me."

"Andre"

Anonymous

Andre was 30 years old the day he noticed his colour was a bit off. I was 30 years old the day, two weeks later, I told him his diagnosis. The ensuing nine months were filled with struggle and pain and yet, looking back, his was a triumphant death.

Adversity had marked much of Andre's life – family troubles, a slightly "wild" youth, and a long struggle with infertility. Finally, at age 30, he had reached a plateau with a valued vocation, loving spouse and adopted family. But now he was ill, off work, and listless. One by one the treatments failed: surgery, then chemotherapy, then the gamut of "alternative therapies." So how would this tragedy be turned to triumph?

Andre's triumph was spiritual. In an age of disbelief he found belief. In a time of hopelessness, he created hope. For his was not the soft spirituality of passivity but rather the solid practical spirituality of facing mortality directly.

From his faith in Christ, Andre was able to summon the resources to deal with his illness and all its ramifications. He communicated his needs to his caregivers without ambiguity. He comforted his diverse family and was able to receive comfort. He lived each day fully and with such determination that even acquaintances were inspired.

To my surprise, I found myself changing through Andre's illness. We became friends, and I began to see myself as his pupil as well. He confirmed that the strategies of palliative care that I had learned, worked well. He affirmed the team approach and gently reminded me of my limitations and needs.

Andre became increasingly ill, and then he died. Some would say that his death is what matters. I would simply reply that Andre lived, and lives on. It is how he lived and how he died that really matters.

"Maxine"

by Kelly Peloquin

At one time I may have viewed this as a non-success story. It was a situation where my need was greater than the patient and her family's needs. In reality, it was a great success and I believe that Maxine's living process until she died was what the family needed as well. There is always room for improvement in any situation and I feel we will learn from the experience.

I initially became involved with Maxine through her course of chemotherapy, in an outreach setting. This was in preparation for her impending bone marrow transplant. She and I went through a lot together. Maxine came through the ordeal fairly well, in my opinion. She felt strongly this was something she had to do despite all the hardships she endured.

To Maxine and her family's horror, the cancer spread to the brain not more than eight months following the bone marrow transplant. This was followed by a course of palliative radiotherapy to help minimize the cancer spreading but this produced only a short period of symptom relief. When she became weaker, and her needs became more than she could handle alone, her strong network of family and friends stepped in and provided a level of home care, meals and tending to the yard that met Maxine's approval. When she was close to death, it was her decision to move to the hospital where she would spend her remaining days.

It was her wish not to die at home where she might ruin it for the rest of the family. There were conflicts between her and her husband that she felt she didn't want to work on even though it would be the last chance. Despite my constant encouragement to resolve these issues it was not her choice. Her family and her friends were there for her to the end. I feel all her wishes were granted even though they were not the same as mine. She said to me, "Not everything turns out perfectly with every family and that is something you have got to understand!"

"Joe"

Anonymous

This is a story of Betty who provided home support to Joe. She became his friend and she reached out to care beyond the responsibilities of her job.

Joe was a 78-year-old bachelor living in a rural Alberta community. He had lived alone all his adult years and had a history of alcoholism. He was diagnosed with terminal cancer of the stomach and began to receive Home Care services. He was a crusty old individual who claimed no one cared about him. Betty was the Home Support worker assigned to provide housekeeping services to Joe. She was very apprehensive, at first, of Joe due to his reputation in the community. However, she began to provide the services and became the most frequent company that Joe had.

As the relationship progressed, Joe indicated a desire to see his sisters once more before he died. He always stated that he had lost touch with them and after all these years they probably wouldn't want to see him anymore. His last contact with family had occurred about forty years ago. While wanting to talk to, and to see his sisters, he was just too frightened of rejection to even start the search.

Betty could see that Joe's health was failing rapidly. Unbeknownst to Joe, she became a "private detective." Joe only knew the province where his sisters had lived and that one had become a nun in the Catholic Church. Betty worked with contacts in the church to obtain possible locations of Joe's sisters. As his condition worsened, Betty started phoning. Miraculously, Betty was able to contact one of the sisters, who knew the location of the other sister as well. When Betty explained about Joe's condition and his whereabouts, they immediately made plans to come to see Joe.

When Betty informed Joe of her actions, he couldn't believe that one human being would care enough about him to do this for him. Joe's sisters were able to visit with him for several days before he died. As he told Betty on the morning of his death, he could die "at peace] because of her actions. "

"Nora"

by Sandra Davies

When I met Nora in 1984 she was living with metastatic ovarian cancer, a mastectomy, a colostomy and monthly debilitating sessions of chemotherapy which left her nauseated and weak for up to four days. She was 64 and had been widowed for five years. Her late, and much beloved, husband had been a member of the lay clergy of the Anglican Church. Her two adopted daughters, survivors of abuse in their early pre-Nora childhood, were grown and married. One lived hundreds of miles away and the other lived in our home town with an alcohol-dependent husband and adolescent children who were in and out of trouble with the authorities. Nora had been an Early Childhood Education graduate and supervisor of a local day care. She was superbly competent in her job and was well loved by staff and by the children for whom she cared.

My job at the time was to "provide palliative care" within: a limited budget, a task-oriented community, and an efficiency-driven, fee-for-visit contracted nursing service. Palliative care was undefined.

Nora taught me most of what I know about palliative care nursing, a course of which I now teach. She was slow to trust and hesitant to share. Some of my colleagues were critical of her needs: "Someone to sit in my bathroom with me twice a week while I soak my damaged body, my raw colostomy, my scarred non-breast; someone to call in the night; someone to promise to keep me clean if I become comatose; someone to tell me when I'm starting to die." None of these were the physical tasks from which my colleagues took comfort. Palliative care was relatively new in our community and its demands were not well understood.

I sat and listened and wept and struggled as Nora carried on, patiently accepting my help and giving me her support. Homemakers were interviewed and dismissed until Dixie arrived and performed loving miracles with tidbits of food, expert plumping of pillows and a shining clean room. More help was needed and the money was running out. Her daughter moved in. "It's time for me to give something back," she said. She learned colostomy care, morphine injection administration, and anti-nausea techniques. I visited twice a day, then three times, and then four. Her doctor was enlisted, sat on her bed, spoke of her dying and of spirituality. The priest came and her grandsons learned to lift her up in bed. The new team of caregivers grew and learned.

Finally, Nora decided to stop her chemotherapy. "I'm ready now, Sandra. Please keep me clean and out of pain. I want a party to say goodbye but we'll pretend it's a birthday party for my granddaughter." Her eyes twinkled. The party was scheduled. Nora got weaker and we moved the party ahead. One day she took my hand, looked me in the eye and dared me to break contact. "I'm dying now, aren't I?" She was so calm! "It would seem so, Nora," I answered and we smiled together. Smiled!

On the day of the party, she asked me to get her dressed in her best outfit. "Only on the top, that's all of me they're going to see." She put on dangling earrings. "Do they make me look like an old scrawny witch? – Then take them off." Her best sheets, flowers and "Kentucky Fried Chicken – my granddaughter's favourite." Then, a satisfied, loving grin – "It's just the way I pictured it!"

The party was bitter sweet and a great success for Nora and her family. And for me. Six days later, Nora died in the company of her loved ones. She was clean and pain free to the end.

"A Success Story: Patient and Volunteers"

by Anne Goertzen

I got the referral from a doctor. The patient had lung cancer and was in the hospital. He used to be a 300-pound man and now was all skin and bones.

I walked to his room to do the assessment. He greeted me very friendly because he had been informed by the doctor that we at the hospital had a palliative care program which he could benefit from. He was very cooperative with the assessment even though he did have shortness of breath at times. He told me about his illness. He also told me about looking for help from different doctors during his illness. We had a nice visit.

I asked him whether he would mind a lady volunteer. He said that was no problem. While doing the assessment I found out that he really liked music. I had a volunteer who plays the harp. I matched him with her and it was a perfect match.

After a while this patient went home. Even though he lived 23 miles out of town this volunteer would visit him quite frequently. The home setting for him was bright. He had a bed in the living room with the window facing the street. People walked in and out. He also was rushed to the hospital quite frequently. The volunteer kept on making her regular visits.

He was admitted to hospital two weeks before his death. A very sick man by then, he needed 24-hour palliative care and he preferred to be in hospital.. This was arranged by the Coordinator together with the family. Nights were very rough on him. At first, he refused volunteers at night. After two very restless nights he agreed he would give it a try. The volunteer sat with him all night and left at 7:00 in the morning. At 8:00 a.m. the coordinator came into his room and he looked so relaxed and with a big smile said, "I did not think it would make such a difference." For seven nights we sat with him.

The last night a good friend of his called. He wanted to stay with him. I told his friend that I would go and ask him. When I came to his bedside, I told him his best friend had called and wanted to stay with him. He refused him. He did not want him to come. He wanted a palliative care volunteer. I called his friend back and he said, "You hurt my feelings." What could I as a coordinator do but accept the patient's wishes?

He died early that morning with the volunteer beside him. His wife and part of the family arrived in time before he died. The family was so grateful for the palliative care volunteers. Some of us attended the funeral which was much appreciated by the family. The bereavement follow-up carried on for five months. After five months, the wife and the two children living with her in their home were ready for a trip to B.C. We closed the case. The wife and one daughter are now regular attenders in a cancer support group.

"Husband, Father, Friend, Farmer"

by Thelma Alexander

My story is about a 53-year-old farmer, with four beautiful daughters, who faced terminal illness by including his family and friends into his personal space.

When he travelled to the city hospital for a lengthy operation no one knew he would not undergo this operation. Instead, after a short exploratory surgery, he was back in his hospital room. The physician explained to his wife that there was nothing that could be done to alleviate the farmer's distress as the cancer had spread. The wife had to explain this to her husband and then to her daughters; two of whom were married and two of whom were college students. No wheelchair was provided when he walked out of his room carrying his personal possessions in the black garbage bag provided.

He returned to his farm, starting proceedings to auction off the machinery and put his affairs in order. He was an excellent craftsman and whenever he noticed that renovations were needed he worked until his strength was exhausted and he could no longer lift the tools required to complete the job.

He made time to speak to each of his daughters, assuring them of his love and telling them of his hopes and dreams for them. The daughters responded by preparing palatable foods, by singing and playing piano selections for him, by massaging his feet, and bringing him cushions to elevate him to more comfortable positions. They took the time to listen and to be with him at every possible moment.

While he was still able, he visited all his friends and when he became unable to travel, he responded to the home care nurses with a courtesy that endeared him to all. His wife cooked food that he could digest and guarded him from over zealous relatives or friends who came to visit during his last days.

He wanted so badly to stay at home that a bed in the sitting room was made for him where he remained until one day before his death. Then the trauma of choking spells increased and finally his wife called for the ambulance. When he entered the hospital she informed the doctor that he was worried he would not get the same treatment that he had received at home. The doctor assured him that they would not change his routine and the family could assist in the hospital as they had done at home.

As a friend, I could only stand in the background and help when I saw a need. What was it that caused me to waken early, bake muffins and venture the eight miles at sun rise to be with a dear friend? When I arrived, preparations were being made to transfer him to the hospital. Just being there as a friend to assist whenever possible was a gift. I whispered in his ear, "We (my family) will help your family in any way we can." We believe that if one truly cares for the deceased, then one will be there for his or her loved ones.

The success in this story is the patient's willingness to accept help, but also to give of his wisdom to friends and family so that even to this day, seven years later, his spirit lives with us.

"Mr. Prumble"

by Dianne A. Hyland

I had only graduated from nursing school less than a year ago when I met Mr. Prumble. He was my mentor from the day we met. He was diagnosed as having early stages of prostrate cancer.

It wasn't long before we realized that his cancer had metastasised and his health was failing. Mr. Prumble, I thought, was a difficult patient. When I came in to give him his bed bath, he would refuse and indicate he wanted it later. He refused to eat when we tried to feed him. He would take off his sanitary products and throw them in the corner. One day, very frustrated, I asked him, "What do you want?" "I want to die with dignity."

This made me stop and realize that he was a human being who could still make his own decisions.

I found out that the reason why he refused his bath was because he was in pain. When I scheduled his bath after the pain medication was administered, it was more comfortable for him.

I began asking him what he wanted to eat for meals. He gave me requests and I even made home-made chicken noodle soup for him. I also respected his wishes when he only wanted sips of water.

By changing his sanitary products more often, I kept him dry and odour free which had really bothered him before.

On my last day of work before going off for a week to get married, I told Mr. Prumble that I would be away. He told me that he would still be here when I got back because he was going to die on my shift. He told me that I should always listen to my patients and go with what is in your heart instead of following the textbook.

I was very angry when I went home. I didn't want anyone to die on my shift. I felt he was getting even with me for all our past confrontations. My fiance said to look at the situation more optimistically.

When I returned to work I learned at report that Mr. Prumble was failing quickly and he hadn't been expected to make it through the night. I quickly went to his room and noticed a drastic change from the week before. I went to his bed and held his hand. I told him I was there with him. His eyes fluttered and he looked at me and said, "Don't be afraid to let your patients die. Just be there for them and respect their wishes." I had tears in my eyes when he told me that someday I would understand. I gave him a kiss and held his hand until he died about an hour later.

Now that I am involved in palliative care I can honestly say that Mr. Prumble had an insight into how I could make a difference in nursing. Thank you, Mr. Prumble.

"Kasey's Success Story"

by Shari Douglas

My hairdresser's father was diagnosed with cancer of the liver. During my appointment she proceeded to tell me about this and how he was coping really well with the news. They had lots of hope and they were gong to fight this – a story we have all heard many times. My job is to develop palliative care policy and programming within my organization and to teach palliative care philosophy to caregivers.

As I began to talk with her about the issues surrounding her father's new diagnosis and how to talk to people with cancer, it became clear that this was not what she wanted or needed from me. My own personal feeling about the situation was one of frustration. My thoughts were, "But I know what is ahead for you and I can help you get through this. I don't want to see you slip through the cracks of our system and suffer unnecessarily." I withdrew and waited but offered to be available at anytime and for any reason.

We had talked briefly in the past about my job and what I do but she clearly didn't understand it and I had received the usual reaction, "You do what?" accompanied by a look of horror.

Over the next few appointments I got a play-by-play description of her father's declining health but he seemed to be doing okay. The family doctor was knowledgeable in pain and symptom control and her father was comfortable. He and the family had worked through many of the issues facing them and had decided that they did not wish hospitalization. He wanted to remain at home to die.

This time I mentioned Home Care and the services available to them. The response was, "Oh no. We can manage. We don't need that." As time passed they did accept a referral and were assessed by the case manager and provided with the supports of their choice and the necessary equipment.

The father was never admitted to hospital at any time during his illness and was treated conservatively as he wished. I might add he had also chosen not to accept any treatment of his illness after being given the information and the options available to him.

After his death, on my next scheduled appointment, Kasey reviewed her experience. She was almost elated and couldn't say enough about their positive experience. She had taken several weeks off work before his death to be with him and to assist her mother in caring for him.

Some of the incidents she recalled were the days when she bathed him and assisted him to use the urinal; the times when she just sat and talked with him for hours. Also the comfortable silent times they shared. She spoke of the time when he was incontinent of stool several times and every time his wife bathed and cleaned him he said, "Honey. You don't have to do this. I'll only mess again in another ten minutes." Her mother replied, "If I'm here and I can do this for you, I want to."

Her father had a habit of winking at his "girls" as he called them. In the final days, he was unable to verbally communicate with them but would still wink when they came into the room. On the day he died, he was semi-comatose due to his liver cancer (not from any of his medications). Kasey and her mother slipped into the room and spoke to him telling him his girls were there. He winked and died peacefully not long after.

Kasey's story of how wonderful this whole experience had been, and how well she and her mother were able to cope following his death, reaffirms my commitment to palliative care and renews my energy to promote and educate so that palliative care is available to all.

* * *

If you, or someone you know, has a palliative care success story, please send it to Harry van Bommel, PSD Consultants, 11 Miniot Circle, Scarborough, Ontario, M1K 2K1. We cannot promise that it will be published in a future edition of this or another book but it will add to the overall data on how successful palliative care can be. There are three main perspectives we are looking for in success stories – the perspectives of people who are dying, their family members and their caregivers.

Part III

The Dorothy Ley Hospice

Recommended Resources

Appendices:

Curriculum Vitae of Dr. Ley

International Work Group on Death, Dying and Bereavement – Statements of Assumptions and Principles

The Dorothy Ley Hospice

The Dorothy Ley Hospice is a tribute to the palliative care philosophy that Dr. Ley worked so hard to help develop and promote in Canada and abroad. It is fitting that we know a little more about this hospice and how it applies the palliative care philosophy to the needs of people who have a terminal or life-threatening illness in the Etobicoke community.

The Dorothy Ley Hospice is a community hospice. There are basically four models of hospice care in Canada: community hospice, free-standing hospice, palliative care unit within a hospital or long-term care facility, and a palliative care team within a health care facility. A community based hospice program has its own Board of Directors and usually serves people who are dying in their own homes. The majority of the services are provided by community volunteers who may be supported by a limited number of paid hospice staff. Community hospices tend to work well with the professional caregivers within the community including the patient's family physician, homecare services and, if necessary, staff at the hospital. The community hospice volunteers may also visit the person who is ill if they are moved to the hospital to provide a continuum of care.

Free-standing hospices, such as Casey House in Toronto or Maison Michel Sarrazin in Sillery Quebec, are separate buildings where people who are dying may go to receive physical, emotional and spiritual supports in their last weeks or months of living. There are only a handful of such free-standing institutions in Canada.

Hospices services within hospitals or long-term care facilities are either separate palliative care units or a team of professionals who will visit patients anywhere within the facility. The choice of which model is used in such facilities is often based on how the service will be funded and how strongly the community demands hospice care. Sometimes, palliative care units are also found in university-teaching hospitals and are, therefore, used to teach physicians, nurses, social workers, chaplains and others about palliative care.

In recent years there has been a trend to combine some of these models of care. Therefore, some hospital-based programs also have a community outreach service that provides services to people in their own homes. As well, some community-based hospices have begun to look at developing free-standing hospices as a further way to meet some of the needs of people who are dying. It is possible that one day one hospice program may provide all these models of care. The great risk is that such a program will become an extension of the traditional health care model which will lead to people who receive services not getting the individualized care that is at the core of the palliative care philosophy.

The Dorothy Ley Hospice in Etobicoke, Ontario is committed to offering support to individuals and their families facing a terminal illness to help them live with comfort, meaning, dignity and hope. All their services are provided without charge. As a community- based organization it is designed to help people remain at home for as long as they choose. The Hospice supports the person who is ill, the family and other caregivers.

The Hospice was initiated by the Outreach Committee of St. George's on-the-Hill Anglican Church in 1985. It was incorporated in 1987 and began serving clients in 1990. Since then, the Hospice has provided support services to more than 300 clients (to the end of 1993). The Hospice is a non-profit organization funded by donations from individuals, churches, service clubs, companies, foundations and bequests. It offers an interdisciplinary team of health care professionals and trained volunteers dedicated to:

- providing high quality care in the home;
- alleviating pain and other symptoms;
- providing assistance with daily activities;
- providing spiritual support through clergy from many different religions with a special interest and training in palliative care;

- collaborating with existing services;
- counselling patients and their families;
- offering support and understanding to the bereaved as long as necessary after the death of a loved one;
- offering educational programs, research opportunities, a newsletter and a speakers' bureau for explaining community hospice care to people in Etobicoke.

In response to a call for assistance, a Hospice team member will visit a patient at home or in the hospital. A personalized care plan is then developed for each patient in consultation with the attending physician, other agencies providing care and the family.

Volunteers receive 30-hours of training provided in collaboration with Humber College in Etobicoke. Men and women of all ages and backgrounds come to the hospice as volunteers. They are provided with ongoing training, education and group support.

For further information you can write or call the hospice at:

P.O. Box 1500 - 401
Etobicoke, Ontario
M9C 4V5
Canada
(416) 255-9500 or 255-7903

Recommended Resources

Aries, Paule. (1951). *The hour of our death.* New York: Knopf.

Buckman, Robert. (1989). *I don't know what to say: How to help and support someone who is dying.* Toronto: Key Porter.

Cassel, Eric J. (1982). The nature of suffering and the goals of medicine, *New England Journal of Medicine*, 306, pp. 639-645.

Corless, I.B. (September 5, 1986). Talk given in New Paltz, New York.

Cousins, Norman. (1979). *Anatomy of an illness.* New York: Norton.

Doyle, Derek; Hanks, Geoffrey W.C.; and MacDonald, Neil. (1993). *Oxford textbook of palliative medicine.* Oxford: Oxford University Press.

Expert Advisory Committee on the Management of Severe Chronic Pain in Cancer Patients. (1984). *Cancer pain: A monograph on the management of cancer pain.* Ottawa: Ministry of Supply and Services.

Feifel, Herman (Ed.). (1977). *New meanings of death.* New York: McGraw-Hill.

Frankl, Viktor. (1987). *Man's search for meaning* (Revised Edition). London: Hodder and Stoughton.

Glebe, Delton. (1990). Spirituality in the grief process, in *Saying goodbye: Essays*. Toronto: TVOntario Publications.

Goldberg, Ivan K., Austin H. Kutscher and Sidney Malitz (Eds.). (1986). *Pain, anxiety and grief: Pharmacotherapeutic care of the dying patient and the bereaved*. New York: Columbia University Press.

International Work Group on Death and Dying and Bereavement. Their publications on death education, and spiritual care of people who are dying and their families.

Koka, Kenneth J. with John D. Morgan. *Death and spirituality*. (1992). Amityville, NY: Baywood Publishing Company, Inc.

Kushner, Harold S. (1981). *When bad things happen to good people*. New York: Schocken Books.

Librach, S. Lawrence. (1991). *The pain manual: Principles and issues in cancer pain management*. Toronto: Pegasus Healthcare.

Lifton, R.J. (1979). *The broken connection*. New York: Simon and Schuster.

Morgan, John D. (Ed.). (1988). Death and bereavement: Spiritual, ethical and pastoral issues, *Death Studies*, Volume 12.

Nouwen, Henri J.M. (1972). *The wounded healer: Ministry in contemporary society*. New York: Doubleday.

Saunders, Cicely (Ed.). (1984). *The management of terminal disease*. London: Edward Arnold (Publishers).

Saunders, Cicely. (1988). Spiritual pain, *Journal of Palliative Care*, 4:3, pp. 29-32.

van Bommel, Harry. (1993). *Choices for people who have a terminal illness, their families and their caregivers* (3rd Edition). Toronto: NC Press.

van Bommel, Harry. (1992). *Dying for care: Hospice care or euthanasia*. Toronto: NC Press.

van Bommel, Harry (1986, 1993). *The learn for yourself self-study series*. Scarborough: PSD Consultants.

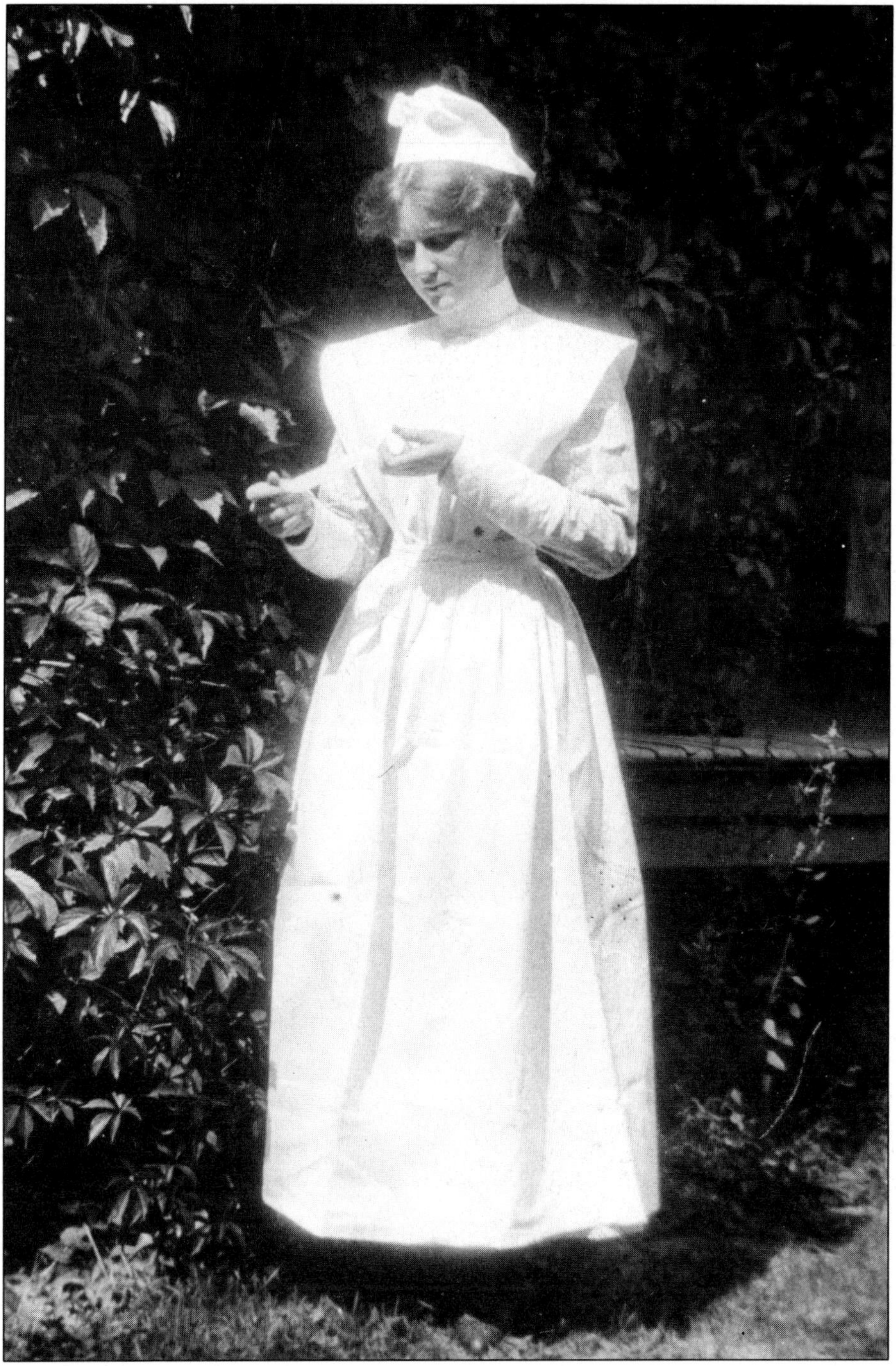

Dorothy's mother, Inez Corinne Dunlop (Ley) in nursing uniform of the early 20th century.

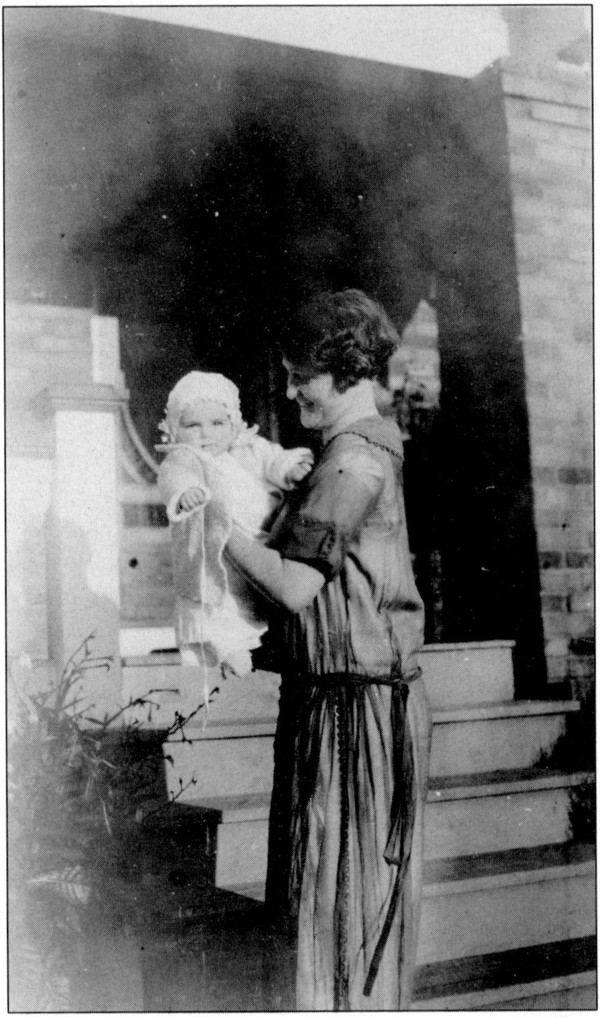

Dorothy and her mother in 1924.

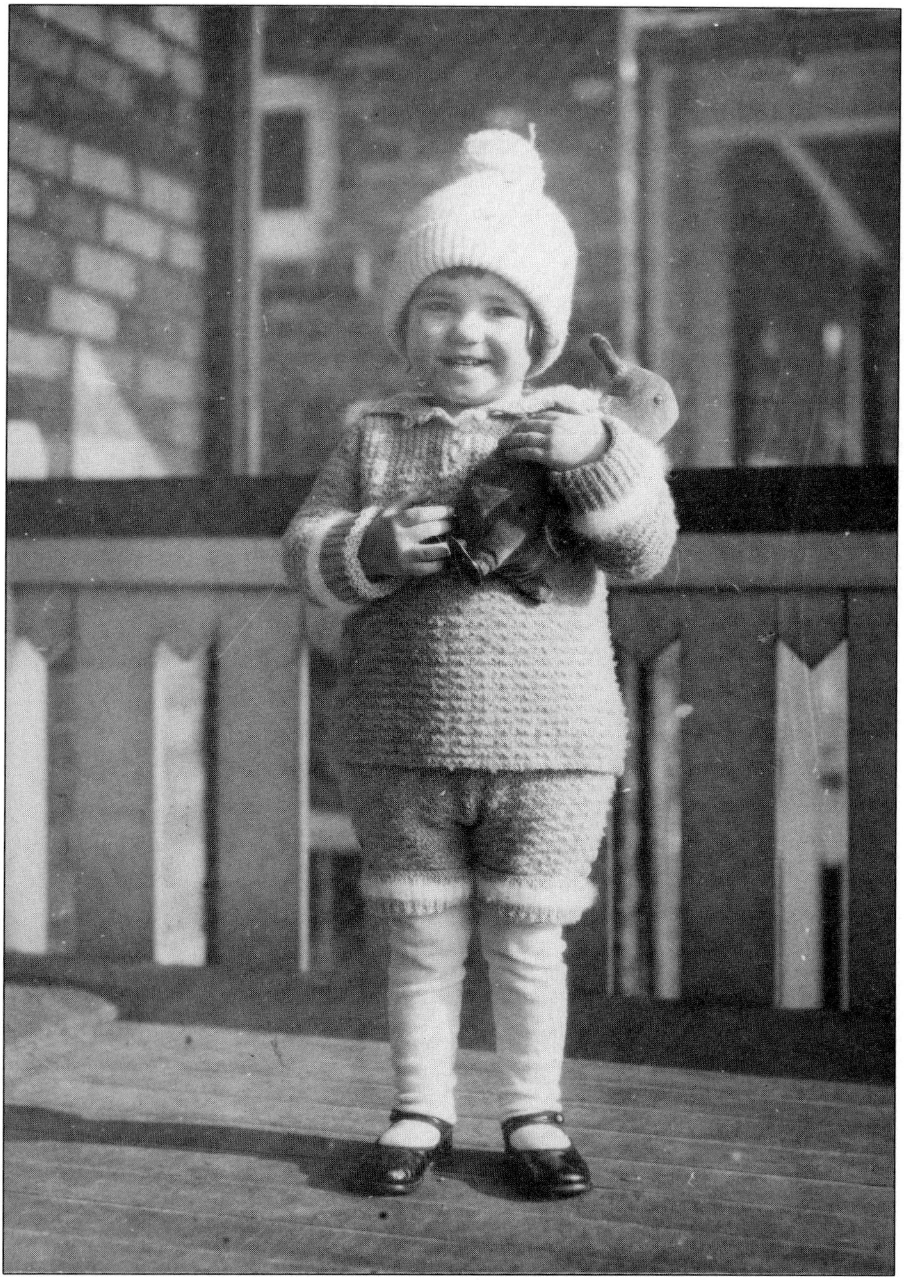

Dorothy with her first collectable bunny (1925 or 1926).

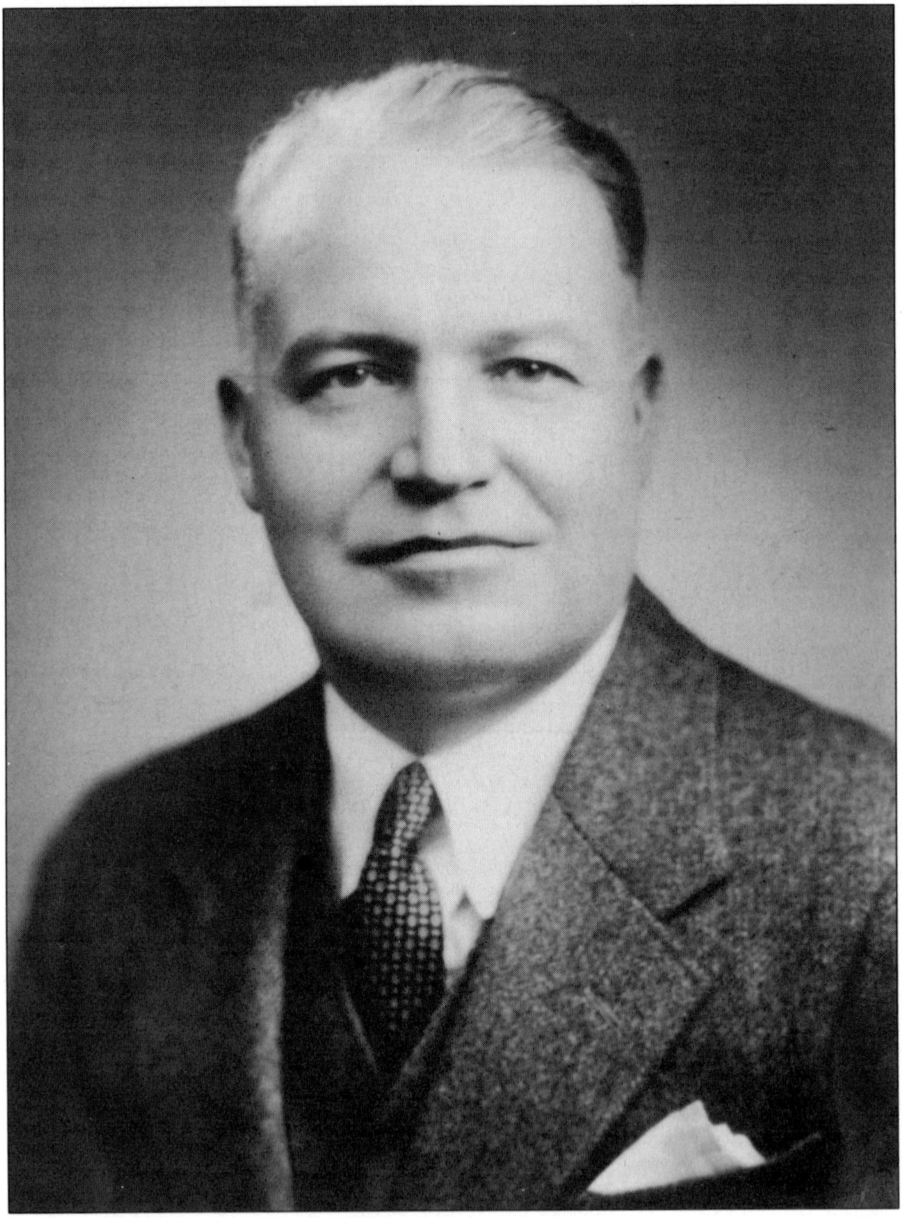

Dorothy's father, Charles Thomas Hobbs Ley.

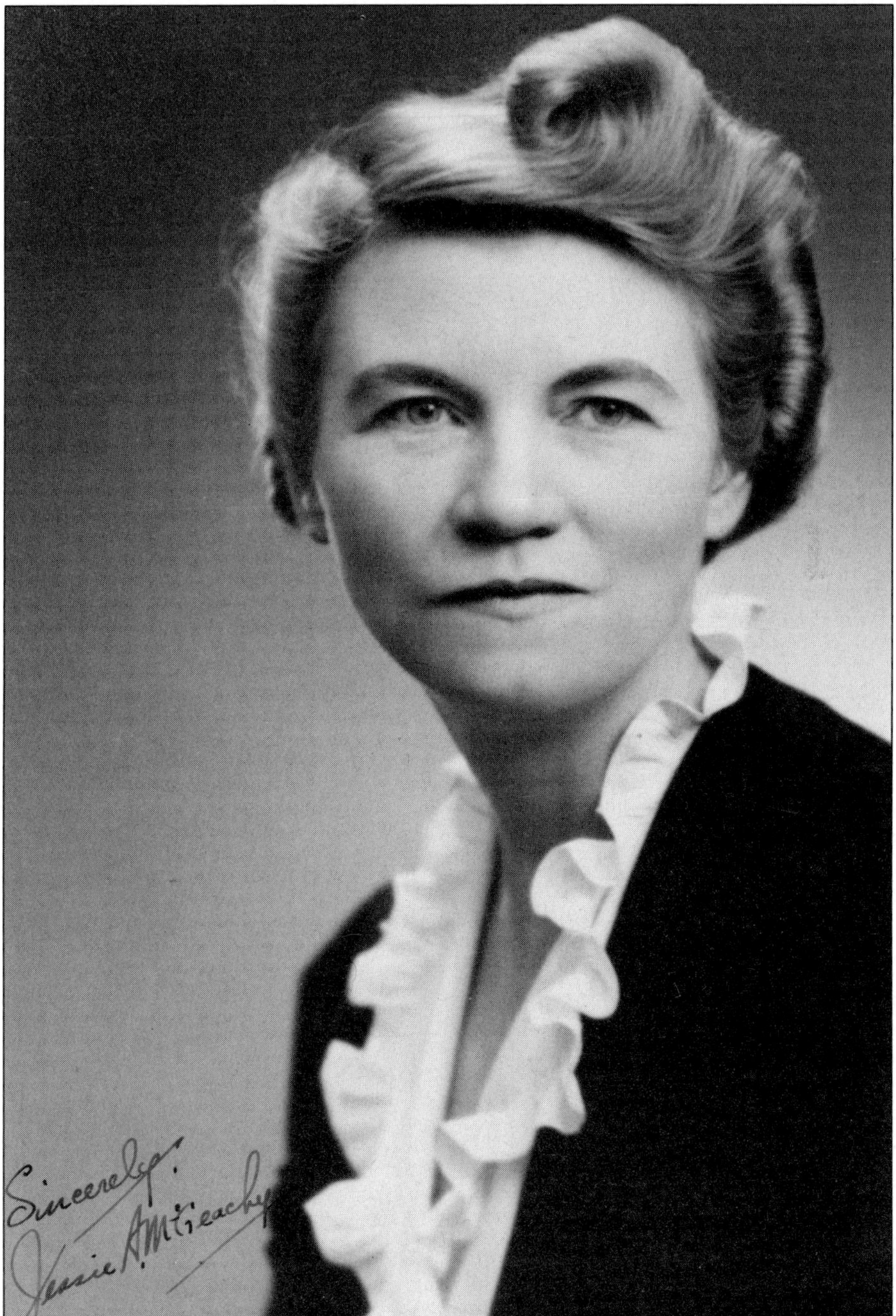

Dr. Jessie McGeachy.

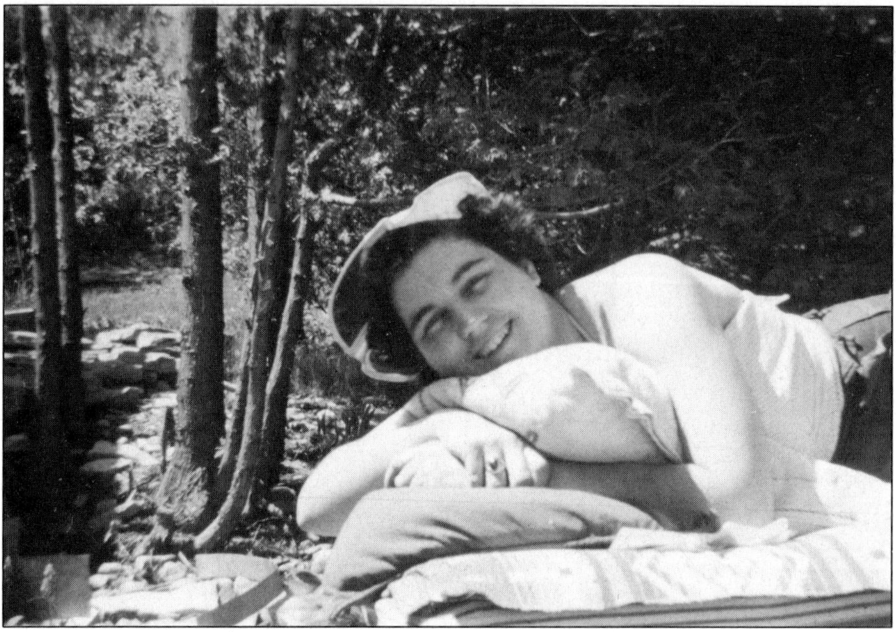

The camper and outdoor enthusiast.

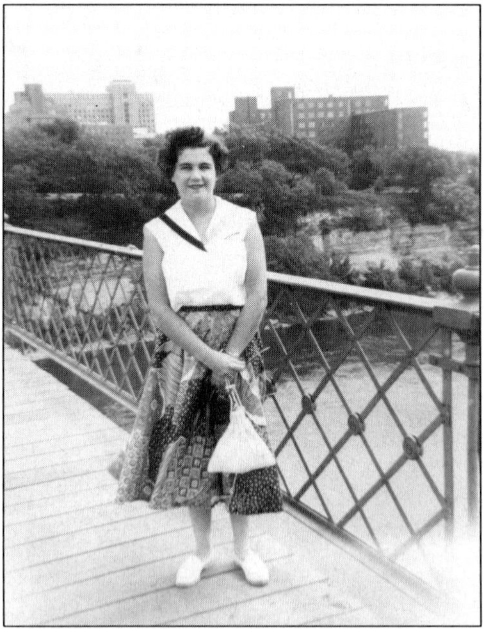

Medical student.

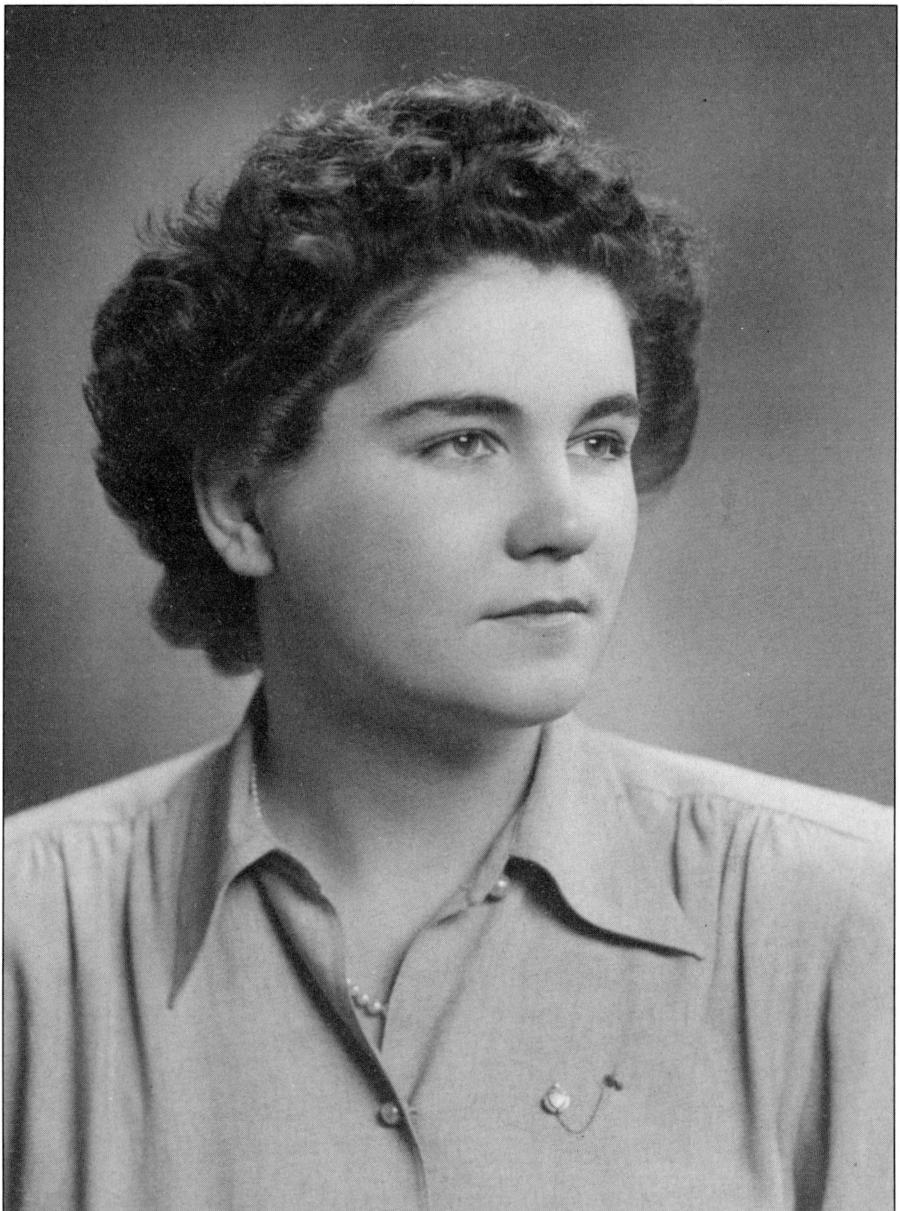

Dorothy in the mid-1940's.

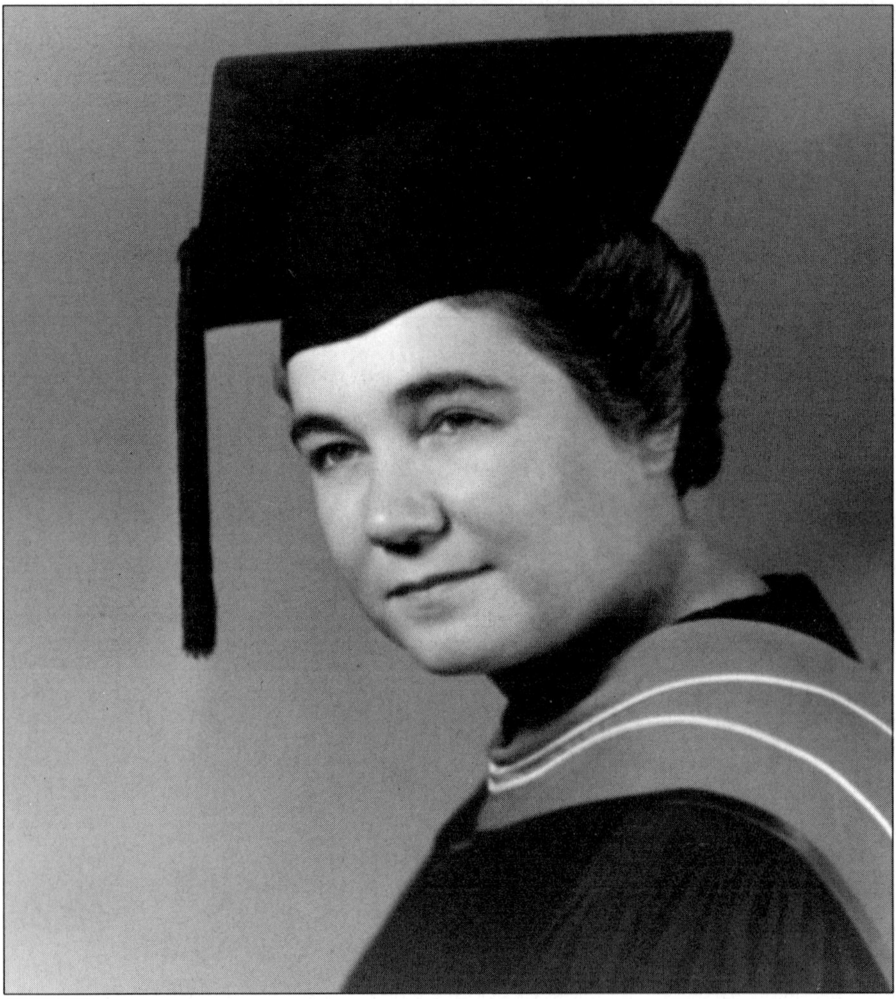

Graduation picture.

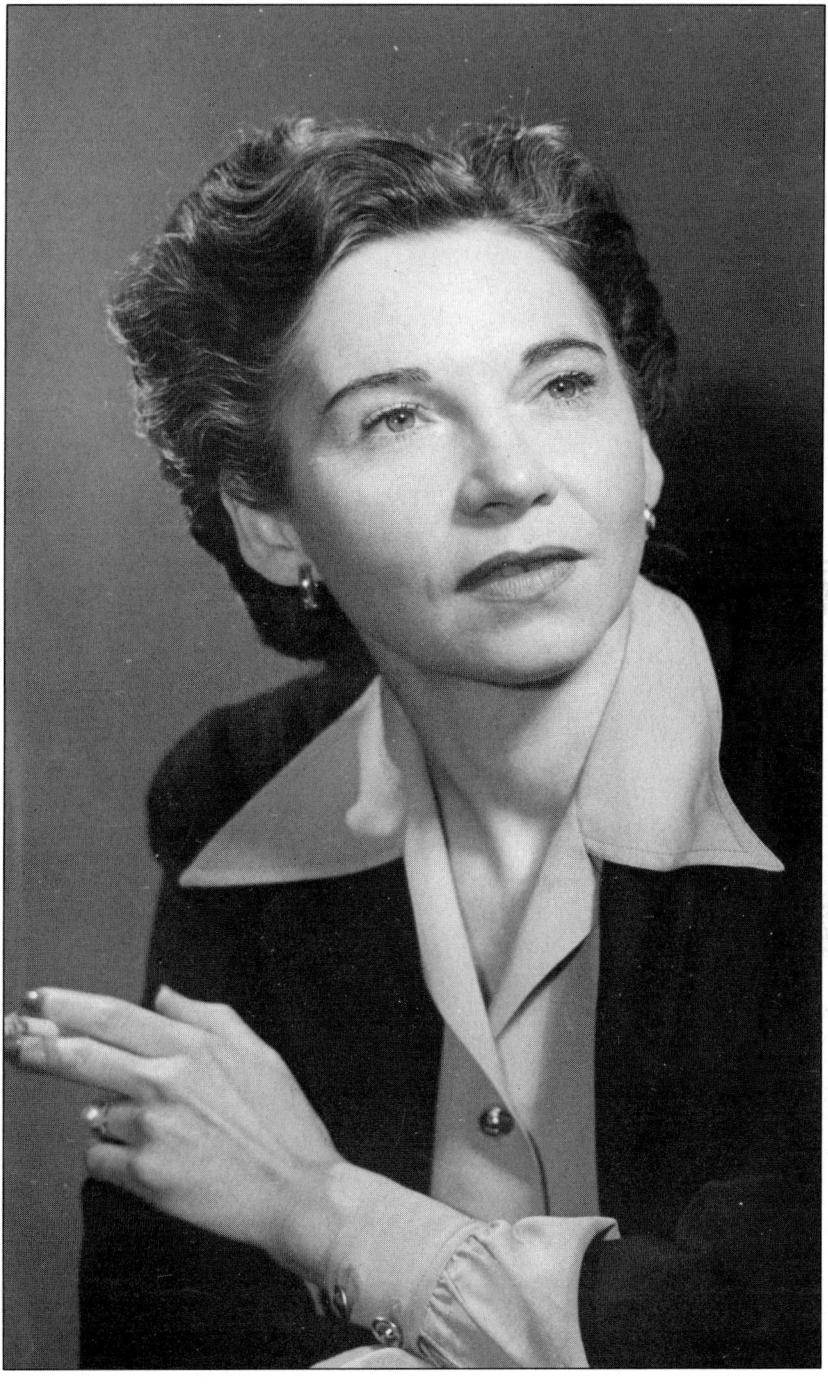

Donnie McGeachy during her acting career in New York.

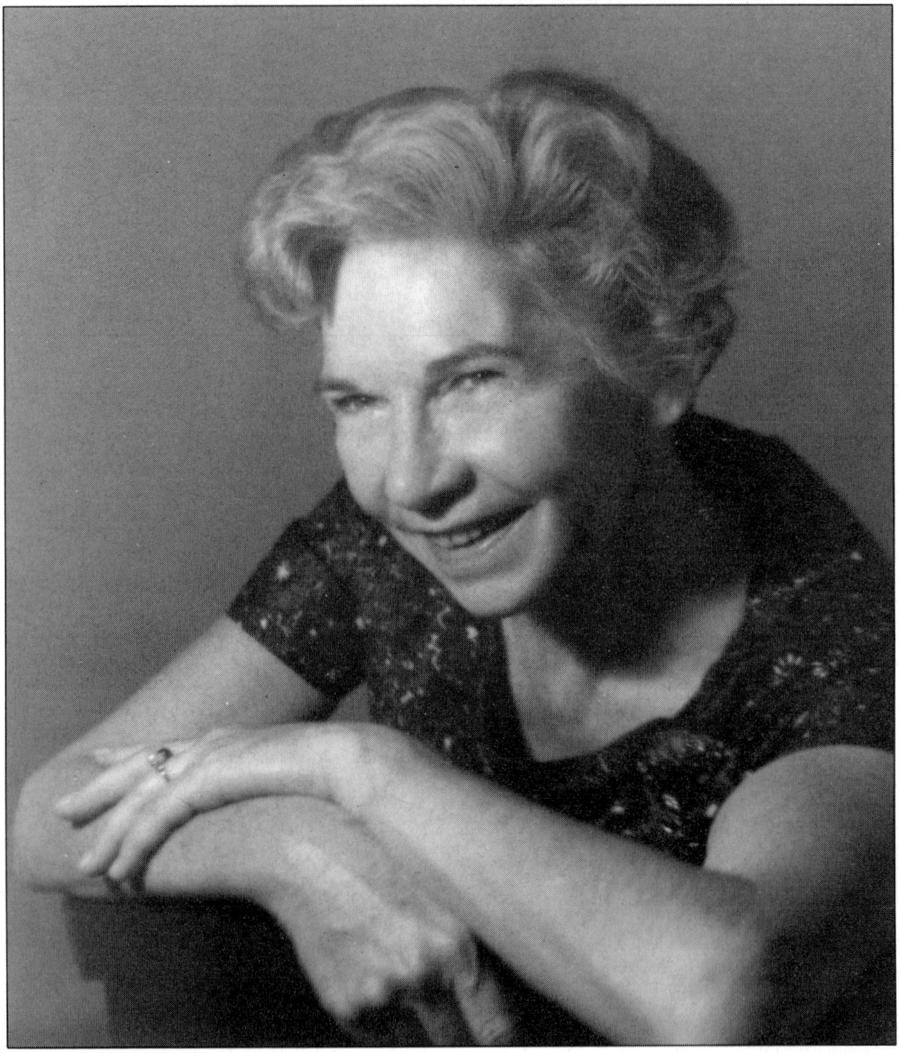

Donnie in her later years.

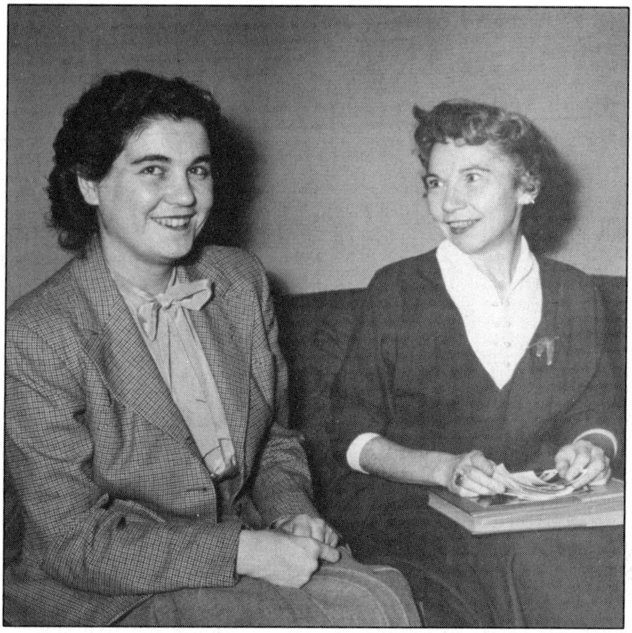

Dorothy and Donnie in the early '50's.

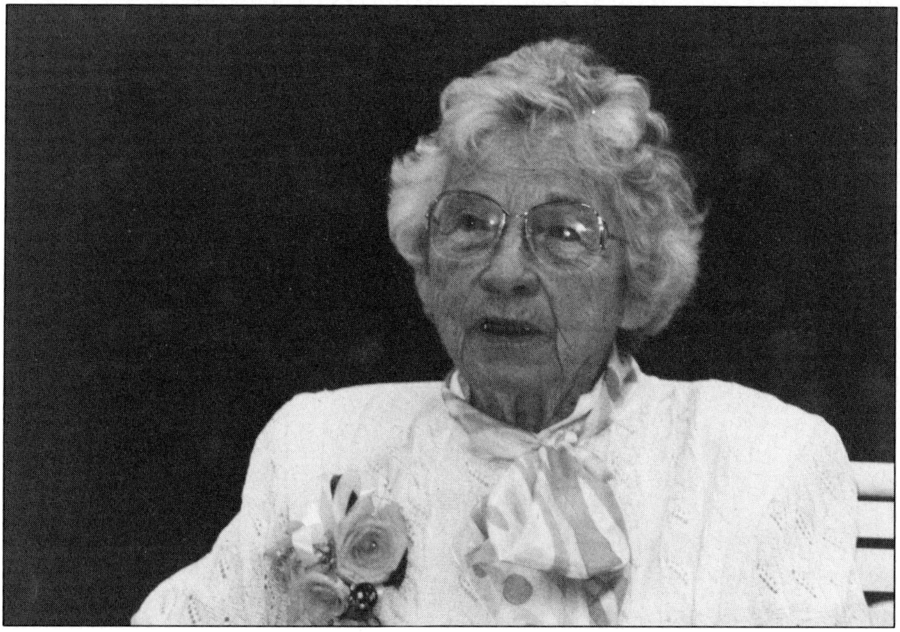

Donnie on her 80th Birthday.

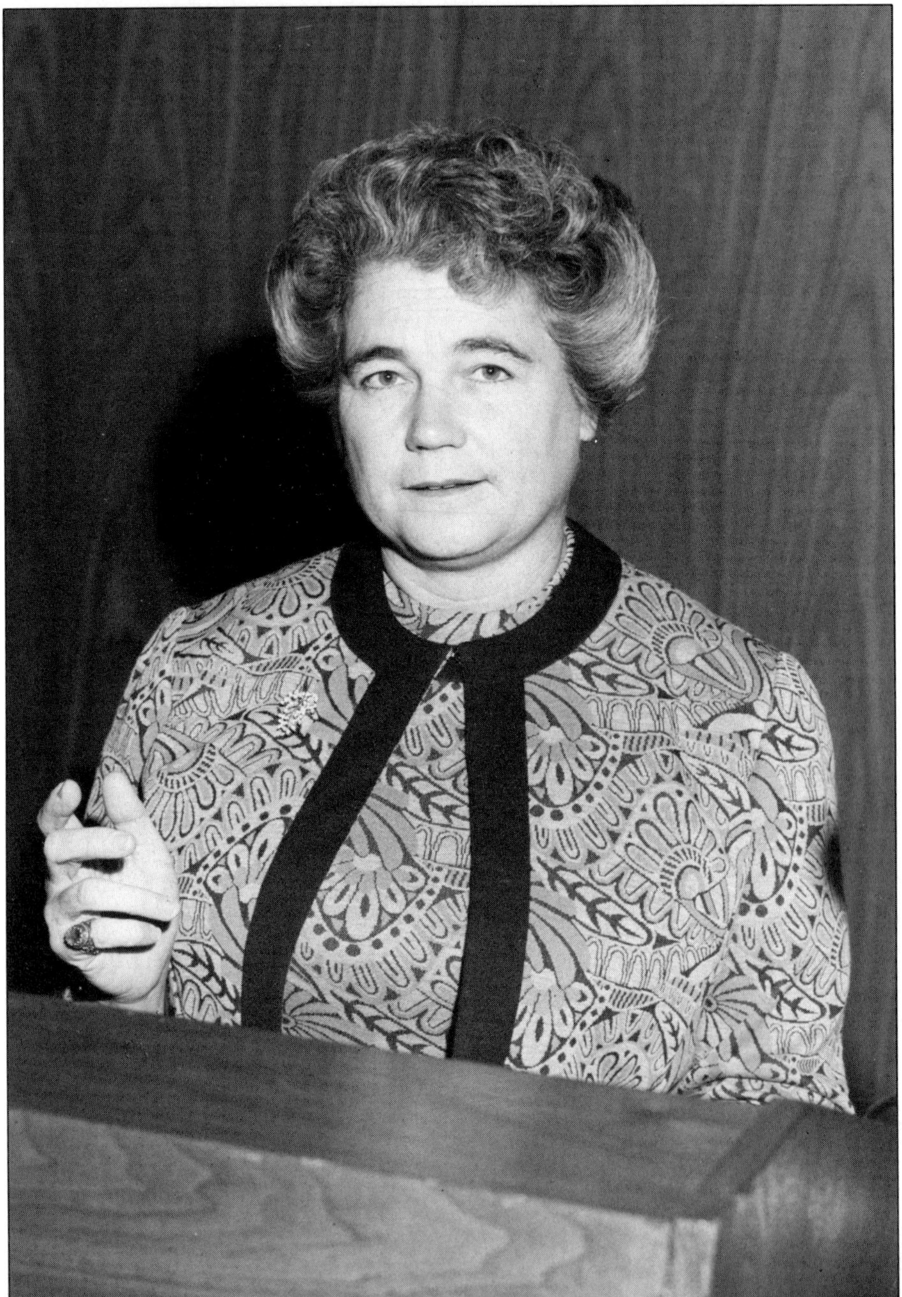

Dorothy giving a medical lecture.

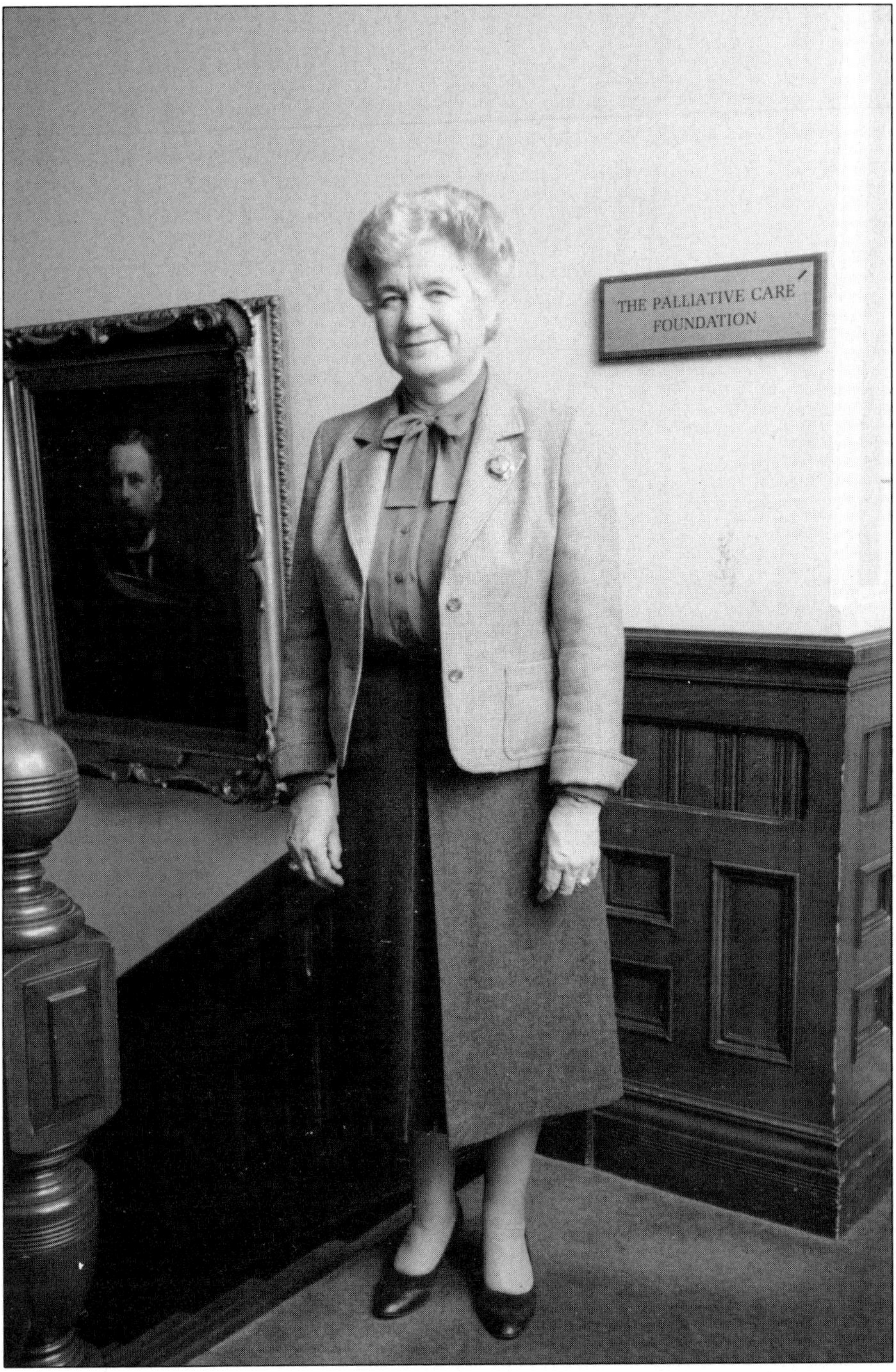

Outside the Palliative Care Foundation office in the early 1980's.

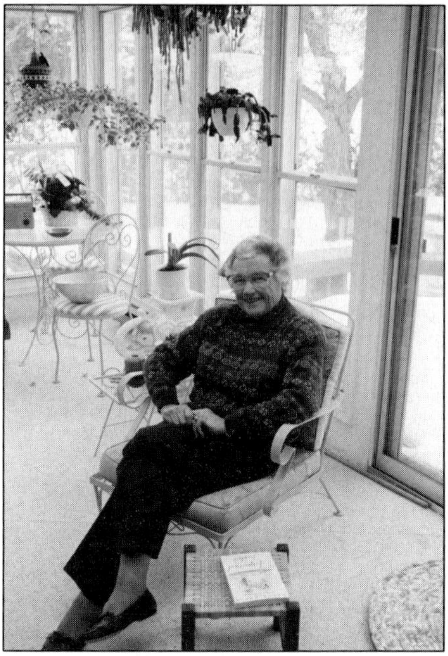

In the sun room at Tir N'an Og.

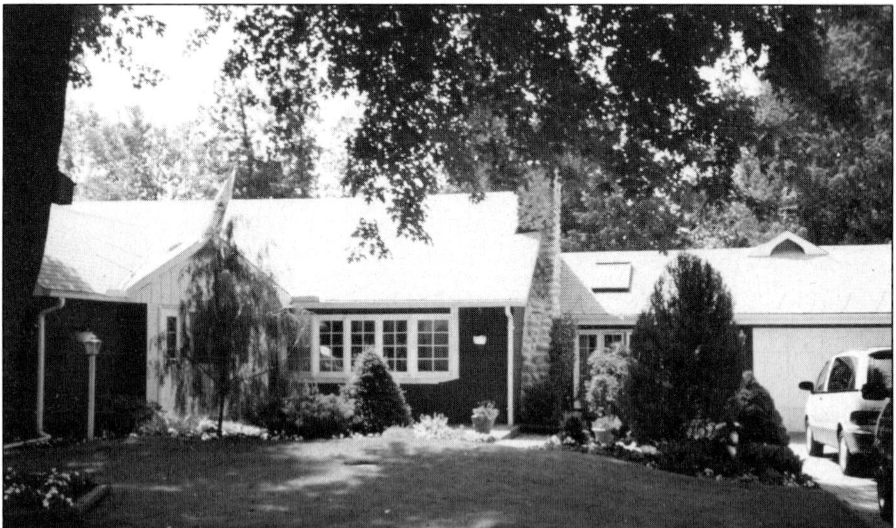

Dorothy's home, Tir N'an Og, on lake Simcoe in Beaverton, Ontario (1992). Photo by Marilyn Lundy.

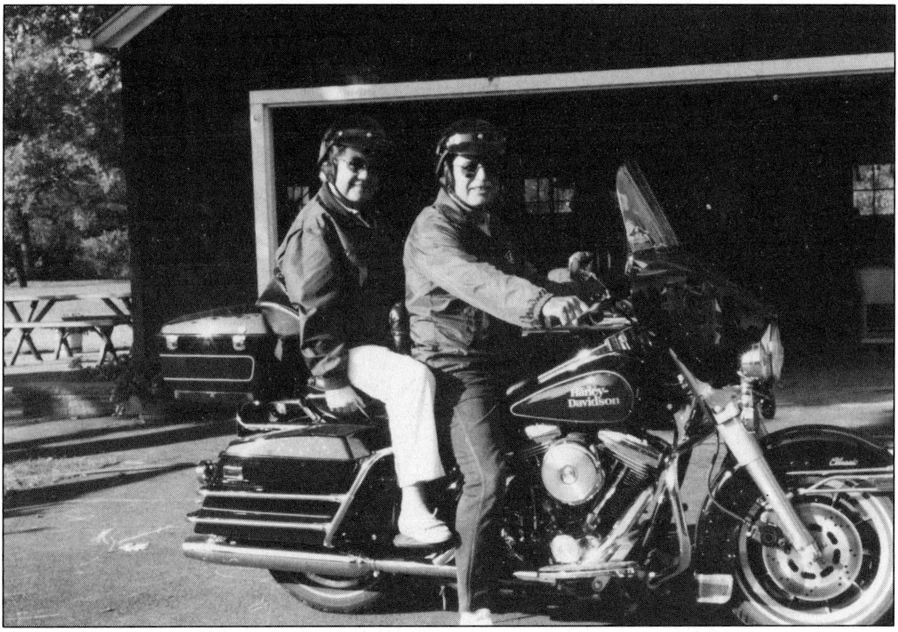

The Doctor and the Judge.

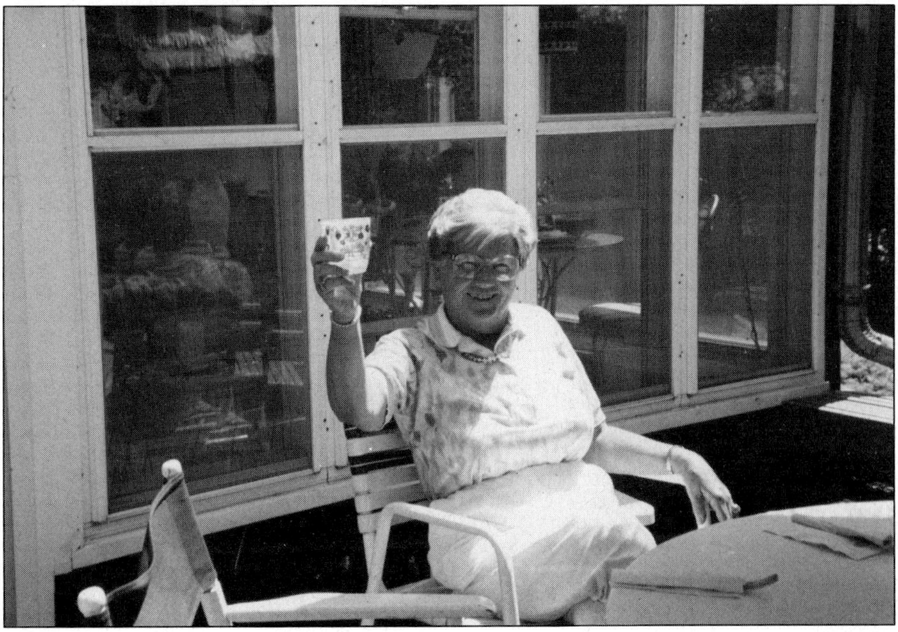

Dorothy in her backyard at Tir N'an Og (1992). Photo by Marilyn Lundy.

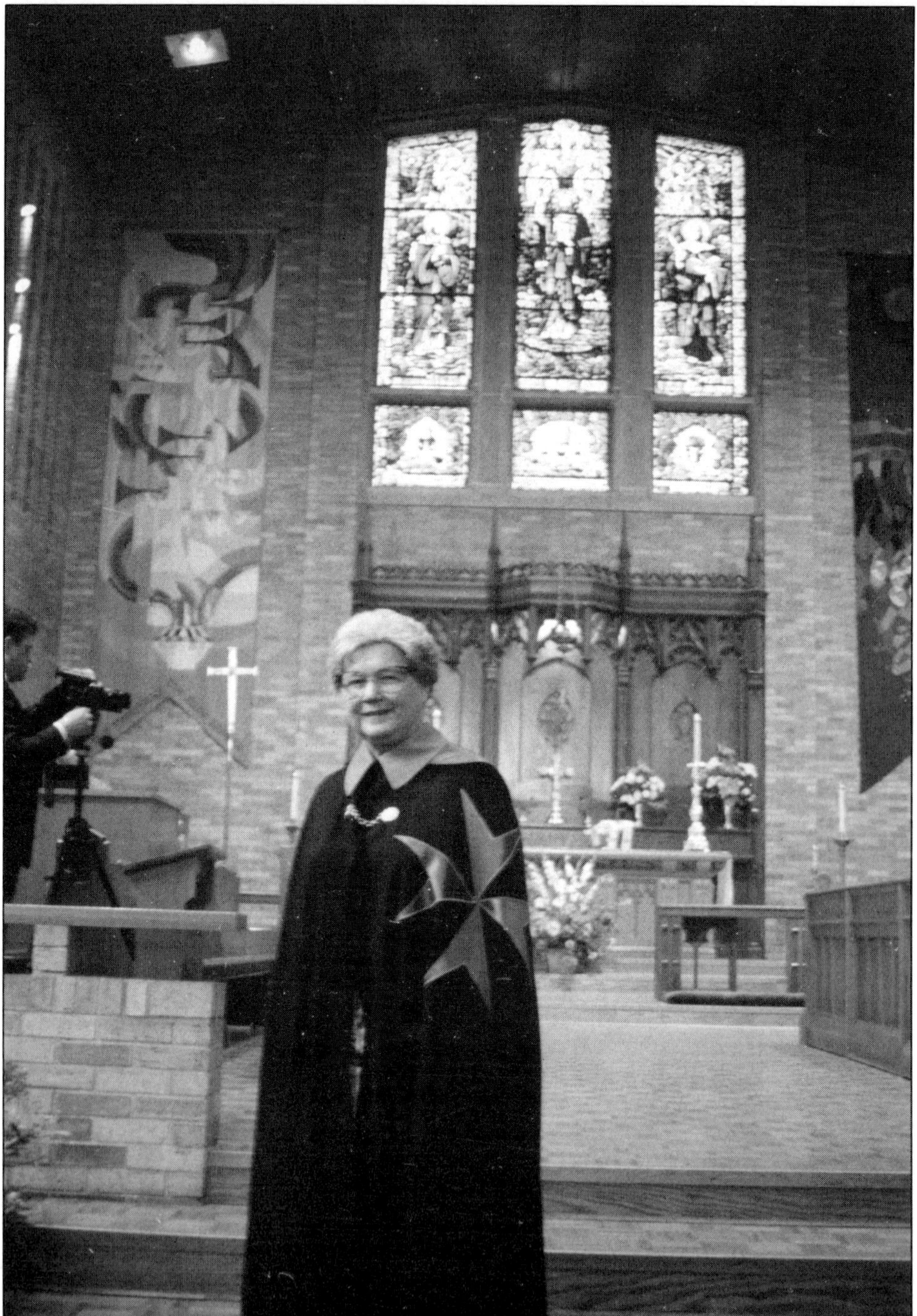

Dame in the Order of St. Lazarus.

Appendix 1:

Cirriculum Vitae

Dr. Dorothy Ley accomplished many things in her life and received many awards in recognition of her contributions to the field of cancer research and practice, as an entrepreneur owning a chain of medical laboratories, as a pioneer in the fields of palliative care, death, dying and bereavement and in the growing area of meeting the needs of our aging population.

She achieved many "firsts" including: first Canadian woman awarded an honourary fellowship of the American College of Physicians, and the first Canadian woman physician to receive the Canadian Medical Association Medal of Service.

Another honour was receiving the Commander of the Order of St. Lazarus (1989) and later becoming a Dame in the same order. This order traces its origin to the Crusades in the 12th century. It is not affiliated with any specific religion today and has branches in countries across the world. Traditionally its reemergence began in France and the modern order's main object was to provide treatment and do research to fight leprosy. It has extended its scope of interests to include other areas of medicine. The order flourished in Quebec during the French regime and was re-established two hundred years later to help further the case of national unity (being the first organization to receive a federal charter in both official languages) and to do charitable work.

Her achievements are highlighted in her curriculum vitae reproduced below.

Education

1936-1941 Lawrence Park Collegiate Institute
1941-1948 University of Toronto

Degrees

1948 Doctor of Medicine, University of Toronto (cum laude)
1951 B.Sc. (Med.) Pathological Chemistry, University of Toronto
1956 Fellow of the Royal College of Physicians (C)
1966 Fellow of the American College of Physicians

Training

1948-1949 Junior Rotating Internship Toronto General Hospital
1949-1950 National Research Council Fellow Department of Pathological Chemistry University of Toronto
1950-1951 Fellow in Pathology: Women's College Hospital and Banting Institute
1952-1953 Senior in Medicine, Ward I, Toronto General Hospital
1953-1954 Assistant Resident in Medicine, Barnes Hospital, Washington University, St. Louis, Missouri
1954-1956 N.R.C. Fellow, Department of Medicine, Toronto Western Hospital
1956-1958 Clinical Research Associate, Ontario Cancer Treatment and Research Foundation, Toronto Western Hospital
1958 Gordon Richards Travelling Fellowship, Canadian Cancer Society

Honour Society

1948 Alpha Omega Alpha Honour Medical Fraternity

Honours

1992 Dame of the Military and Hospitaller Order of Saint Lazarus of Jerusalem

1989 Commander of the Military and Hospitaller Order of Saint Lazarus of Jerusalem

1989 Neville Hodson Walker Award, Metropolitan Toronto District of the Ontario Medical Association for "service, selflessness and sacrifice in the field of medicine and her outstanding contribution as a doctor"

1988 Medal of Service, Canadian Medical Association (1st woman so honoured)

1980 Listed in *Who's Who of American Women*

1977 Her Majesty's Jubilee Medal

1963 Certificate of Merit, Canadian Cancer Society

No dates: Life Member of the International Council of Women Senior Member, Canadian Medical Association Life Member of the Ontario Medical Association

Research

Iron Metabolism Alternation in blood chemistry and haematology in malignant disease; cancer chemotherapy – clinical trials and evaluation.

Appointments

Attending Physician, Toronto Western Hospital (1956-1972)

Director of Haematology and of the Tumour Clinic, Toronto Western Hospital

Assistant Professor of Medicine, University of Toronto Faculty of Medicine (1967-1972)

Director (and designer), Laboratory Proficiency Testing Program, Section on Laboratory Medicine, Ontario Medical Association

Consultant to Clinical Laboratories, Oakville-Trafalgar Memorial Hospital

Founder and President, Toronto Medical Laboratories Ltd. (now part of MDS Health Group)

Past President, Academy of Medicine, Toronto (1975-1976)

Past Chairman, Quality Control Committee Intersociety Council of Laboratory Medicine of Canada

Member, National Survey of Palliative Care Programs in Canada
Founder, President and CEO of the Palliative Care Foundation (1981- 1986)
Founder, Canadian Conference of Palliative Care (held every 2 years)
Member of the Executive Committee, Casey House Hospice, Toronto (1986-1988)
Lay Reader and Warden, Anglican Church of Canada
Parish Representative to the Provincial and Diocesan Synods, Anglican Church of Canada
Member, Church Development Board, Diocese of Toronto, Anglican Church of Canada (1986-1987)
Chairman, Canadian Medical Association Committee on the Health Care of the Elderly (1984-1987)
Chairman, President's Special Committee for Implementation of the CMA Report on Health Care of the Elderly
Canadian Representative to the World Council of Churches Consultation on AIDS in Tanzania, 1989
Canadian Representative to the Board of Directors of the National Hospice Organization of the United States of America
Vice-Chairman, Board of Directors, International Work Group on Death, Dying and Bereavement
Vice-Chairman, Annual Meeting Scientific Planning Committee, Ontario Medical Association
Member, Professional Services Committee, Victorian Order of Nurses for Canada
Member, Board of Directors, York Region Branch, Victorian Order of Nurses
Member, College of Bishops Task Force on AIDS, Diocese of Toronto, Anglican Church of Canada
Member, Board of Directors and Health Services Advisory Committee, Casey House Hospice, Toronto
Chairman, Quality Assurance Sub-Committee, Health Services Advisory Committee, Casey House Hospice
Member, Executive, Ontario Medical Association Section on Palliative Care

Chairman, Education Sub-Committee of Ontario Medical Association Section on Palliative Care
Member of the Ontario Medical Association Advisory Group on the Elderly.
Chairman, Canadian Coalition on Medication Use in the Elderly.
Chairman, National Continuing Care Liaison Committee.
Canadian Medical Association representative to the National Action Committee of the CNIB re: Blind and Visually Impaired Seniors.
Chairman of the Board and President, The Dorothy Ley Hospice, Toronto.
Chairman, AIDS Committee, Anglican Diocese of Toronto.
Chairman of the Planning Committee, Anglican Diocese of Toronto
Member of the Planning and Development Board, Anglican Diocese of Toronto
Member of the Board of Directors, VON Durham
Member of the Pension Board and Pension Committee, Anglican Church of Canada
Member of the Hospice Durham Steering Committee
Chairman, Metropolitan Toronto District Health Council Task Force on Palliative Care
Past President and Chairman of the Planning Committee, Cedarhurst Golf Club, Beaverton, Ontario
Past President, Beaverton-Thorah Homeowners' Association
Numerous honourary positions with hospice care groups.

Publications

(1994). *The Heart of Hospice*. Toronto: NC Press.
(1992). Spiritual Care in Hospice in *Death and Spirituality*, ed. K. J. Doka and John Morgan.
(1990). Palliative Care (Chapter 7) and The Future of Palliative Care (Chapter 8) in *Saying Goodbye: Essays*. Toronto: TVOntario.

(1989). The Elderly and Palliative Care in *Journal of Palliative Care*, 5:4, 43-58.

(1988). The Casey House Model in *Journal of Palliative Care*, 4:4, 111-115.

(March, 1988). Ethical Issues in Geriatrics: Editorial in *Synapse*, Vol. 4, No. 1.

(1988). Spirituality and Hospice Care: with Corless, Inge B., in *Death Studies*, Vol. 12, No. 2.

(1988). AIDS in Canada, in *AIDS: Principles, Practices and Politics*. Eds: Coreless, Inge B. and Pittman-Lindemann, Mary. Washington, DC: Hemisphere Publishing Corporation.

(April, 1987). *AIDS: Proceedings of the North American Conference on Care of Terminally Ill Persons with AIDS*, Ottawa, Canada. Editor.

(1987). *The Elderly – Challenges for Today – Options for Tomorrow: Report of the Committee on Health Care of the Elderly*. Ottawa: Canadian Medical Association.

(January, 1987). The Problem of Pain, in *Canadian Family Physician*, Vol. 33.

(December, 1986). The Elderly in Canada: Today and Tomorrow, in *Canadian Family Physician*, Vol 32, 2572.

(1986). Heroin – The Next Step, in *Journal of Palliative Care*, 1:2, 46-47.

(1985). Palliative Care in Canada: The First Decade and Beyond, in *Journal of Palliative Care*, 1:1, 32-35.

(November, 1982). Palliative Care Foundation: Source of Support and Help, in *Ontario Medical Review*.

(1980). Proficiency at Hemoglobinometry in Ontario Laboratories Between 1974 and 1979, in *CMAJ*, Vol. 125, 180-181.

(1980). A System of Proficiency Testing in Immunohaematology, in *Clinical Laboratory Haematology*, Vol. 3, 125, 180-181.

(1977). Quality Control in Canada. Editor of *Report of the Intersociety Council of Laboratory Medicine of Canada*. Presented to Health and Welfare Canada.

(1974). Dehydration, in *Encyclopedia Britannica*, Edition 15, 560.

(September, 1974). The Development of an Interlaboratory Proficiency Testing Program for the Province of Ontario: I. A Preliminary Survey of Clinical Chemistry; II. Design of Performance Graphs, in *Clinical Biochemistry*, Vol. 7, 223-238, 239-250.

(May-June, 1973). The Case for Quality Control: Some Comments on Quality Control, Proficiency Testing and Laboratory Licensing, in *Newsletter*, Ontario Society of Medical Technologists.

(October, 1973). *Quality Control in the Routine Laboratory.* For Department of Public Health, Nova Scotia.

(June, 1967). The Use of Nitrogen Mustard for Prevention of Bladder Tumour Recurrence: (with Drs. P. Crassweller and G. Rankin) in *The Journal of Urology*, Vol. 100.

(September, 1966). Thynoma and Erythroid Hypoplasia with Carcinoma of the Pancreas, Bronchiolar Hyperplasia and Pulmonary Tuberculosis, in *Annals of Internal Medicine* (with M. Lipa), Vol. 65, No. 3, 541.

(August, 1964). Preliminary Report on an Iron-Sorbitol-Citric Acid Complex (Jectofer), A New Intramuscular Iron Preparation, in *CMAJ*, Vol. 91, 289-292.

(December, 1963). Current Concepts of Iron Metabolism, in *CMAJ*, Vol 89, 1196.

(November, 1963). Current Concepts of Iron Metabolism, in *CMAJ* (Editorial), Vol. 89.

(October 1963). Mast Cell Disease, in *CMAJ*, Vol. 89, 770-775.

(February, 1962). A Preliminary Report on the Use of 5-Fluoracil in Malignant Disease, in *CMAJ*, Vol 86, 207-210.

(June, 1960). Iron Metabolism in Malignant Diseases: Serum Iron and Iron-Binding Capacity in a Control Group of Hospitalized Patients, in *Applied Therapeutics.*

(May, 1957). Changes in White Blood Cell and Bone Marrow Morphology and Serum Protein Fractions in Induced and Spontaneous Hypersensitivity States, in *The Journal of Allergy*, Vol 28, No. 3, 220-228.

(September, 1957). Radioisotopes in Haematology, in *Modern Medicine of Canada*, 69-78.

Appendix 2:

Statement of Assumptions and Principles

Dr. Dorothy C. H. Ley was a member of the International Work Group on Death, Dying and Bereavement (IWG). As a member she was involved in writing three documents related to this topic: Assumptions and Principles of Spiritual Care (1989), A Statement of Assumptions and Principles Concerning Education About Death, Dying and Bereavement (1992), and A Statement of Assumptions and Principles Concerning Education About Death, Dying and Bereavement for Professionals in Health Care and Human Services (1991). Below are complete texts of these documents. Dr. Ley believed these documents were extremely important and required reading for people involved in providing spiritual care and those involved in providing education on dying, death and bereavement.

The IWG is composed of clinicians, researchers and educators dedicated to the development of research, knowledge and practice dealing with death, dying and bereavement, and with its education. It was founded in 1974 at Columbia, Maryland and includes members (by invitation only) from Australia, Canada, Columbia, France, Germany, Greece, Africa, the United Kingdom and the United States of America. It meets every 18 months in different cities around the world.

The International Work Group has kindly consented for us to reproduce these documents, in their entirety, here. Dr. Ley strongly recommended that readers get their publication, Statements on Death, Dying and Bereavement (1994), edited by Charles A. Corr, John D. Morgan and Hannelore Wass. This book includes the three documents in this appendix but also seven others on: underlying standards of care for the terminally ill; palliative care for children; concerning care for persons affected by HIV Disease; psychosocial care of dying persons and their families; bereavement; care of the dying and bereaved in developing countries; and education about life-threatening illness, death, dying and bereavement for volunteers and non-professionals.

For further information contact the International Work Group Secretariat, King's College, 266 Epworth Avenue, London, Ontario, Canada N6A 2M3 (Tel: 519-432-7946).

The following statements use assumptions and principles based on the following definitions:

Assumption: *A statement accepted as fact on the basis of commonly observed experience.*

Principle: *A collective judgement as to the proper response to the assumption.*

Assumptions and Principles of Spiritual Care

Developed by the Spiritual Care Work Group of the International Work Group on Death, Dying and Bereavement.

Our thanks to the members of the IWG on Death, Dying and Bereavement and the participants of the Sixth World Conference on the Terminally Ill for their helpful comments on earlier versions of this document.

Introduction

In those areas of the world where medical care has been shaped by sophisticated technologies and complicated health care delivery systems, efforts to humanize patient care are essential if the integrity of the human being is not to be obscured by the system. This is especially needed for individuals with chronic maladies or those in the process of dying.

Dying is more than a biological occurrence. It is a human, social and spiritual event. Too often the spiritual dimension of patients is neglected. The challenge to the health care provider is to recognize the spiritual component of patient care and to make resources available for those individuals who wish them and in the form desired.

Spirituality is concerned with the transcendental, inspirational and existential way to live one's life as well as, in a fundamental and profound sense, with the person as a human being. The search for spirituality may be heightened as one confronts death. This uniquely human concern is expressed in a variety of ways both formal and informal. Those who provide care for dying persons must respect each person's spiritual beliefs and preferences and develop the resources necessary to meet the spiritual needs of patients, family members and staff. These resources and associated support should be offered as necessary throughout the bereavement period.

While the modern hospice movement has arisen within Western Society with its particular cultural, social and spiritual milieu, the following principles may be applicable in and adapted to other countries and cultures. Ultimately the Assumptions and Principles of Spiritual Care should influence other aspects of health care and be integrated into the larger system. Their need and manner of implementation, however, will be shaped by the spiritual life of a given individual and society.

GENERAL

ASSUMPTIONS	PRINCIPLES
1. Each person has a spiritual dimension.	1. In the total care of a person, his or her spiritual nature must be considered along with the mental, emotional and physical dimensions.
2. A spiritual orientation influences mental, emotional and physical responses to dying and bereavement.	2. Caregivers working with dying and bereaved persons should be sensitive to this interrelationship.
3. Although difficult, facing terminal illness, death and bereavement can be a stimulus for spiritual growth.	3. Persons involved in this circumstances may wish to give spiritual questions time and attention.
4. In a multicultural society a person's spiritual nature is expressed in religious and philosophical beliefs and practices which differ widely depending upon one's race, sex, class, religion, ethnic heritage and experience.	4. No single approach to spiritual care is satisfactory for all in a multicultural society; many kinds of resources are needed.

5. Spirituality has many facets. It is expressed and enhanced in a variety of ways both formal and informal, religious and secular, including, but not limited to: symbols, rituals, practices, patterns and gestures, art forms, prayers and meditation.

5. A broad range of opportunities for expressing and enhancing one's spirituality should be available and accessible.

6. The environment shapes and can enhance or diminish one's spirituality.

6. Care should be taken to offer settings which will accommodate individual preference as well as communal experience.

7. Spiritual concerns often have a low priority in health care systems.

7. Health care systems presuming to offer total care should plan for and include spiritual care as reflected in a written statement of philosophy, and resources of time, money and staff.

8. Spiritual needs can arise at any time of the day or night, any day of the week.

8. A caring environment should be in place to enhance and promote spiritual work at any time not just at designated times.

9. Joy is part of the human spirit. Humour is a leaven needed even, or especially, in times of adversity or despair.

9. Careivers, patients and family members should feel free to express humour and to laugh.

INDIVIDUAL AND FAMILY (natural and acquired)

10. Human beings have diverse beliefs, understandings and levels of development in spiritual matters.

10. Caregivers should be encouraged to understand various belief systems and their symbols as well as to seek to understand an individual's particular interpretation of them.

11. Individuals and their families may have divergent spiritual insights and beliefs. They may not be aware of these differences.

11. Caregivers should be aware of differences in spirituality within a family or close relationship and be alert to any difficulties which might ensue.

12. The degree to which the patient and family wish to examine and share spiritual matters is highly individual.

12. Caregivers must be non-intrusive and sensitive to individual desires.

13. Health care institutions and professionals may presume they understand, or may ignore, the spiritual needs of dying persons.	13. Spiritual needs can only be determined through a thoughtful review of spiritual assumptions, beliefs, practices, experiences, goals and perceived needs with the patient, or family and friends.
14. People are not always aware of, nor are able, nor wish to articulate spiritual issues.	14. (1) Caregivers should be aware of individual desires and sensitive to unexpressed spiritual needs. (2) Individuals need access to resources and to people who are committed to deepened exploration of and communication about spiritual issues.
15. Much healing and spiritual growth can occur in an individual without assistance. Many people do not desire or need professional assistance in their spiritual development.	15. Acknowledgments and support, listening to and affirming an individual's beliefs or spiritual concerns should be offered and may be all that is needed.
16. Patients may have already provided for their spiritual needs in a manner satisfactory to themselves.	16. The patient's chosen way of meeting spiritual needs should be honoured by the caregivers.
17. The spiritual needs of dying persons and their families may vary during the course of the illness and fluctuate with changes in the physical symptoms.	17. Caregivers need to be alert to the varying spiritual concerns that may be expressed directly or indirectly during different phases of illness.
18. Patients and their families are particularly vulnerable at the time of impending death.	18. Caregivers should guard against proselytising for particular types of beliefs and practices.
19. As death approaches, spiritual concerns may arise which may be new or still unresolved.	19. (1) Caregivers should be prepared to work with new concerns and insights, as well as those which are longstanding. (2) Caregivers must recognize that not all spiritual problems can be resolved.
20. Spiritual care of the family may affect the dying person.	20. Spiritual care of family and friends is an essential component of total care for the dying.

21. The family's need for spiritual care does not end with the death of the patient.

21. Spiritual care may include involvement by caregivers in the funeral and should be available throughout the bereavement period.

CAREGIVERS

22. Caregivers, like patients, may have or represent different beliefs as well as different spiritual or religious backgrounds and insights.

22. Caregivers have the right to expect respect for their belief systems.

23. Many health care workers may be unprepared or have limited personal development in spiritual matters.

23. (1) Staff members should be offered skilfully designed opportunities for exploration of values and attitudes about life and death, their meaning and purpose.

(2) Caregivers need to recognize their limitations and make appropriate referrals when the demands for spiritual care exceed their abilities or resources.

24. The clergy is usually seen as having primary responsibility for the spiritual care of the dying.

24. Caregivers should be aware that they each have the potential for providing spiritual care, as do all human beings, and should be encouraged to offer spiritual care to dying patients and their families as needed.

25. Caregivers may set goals for the patient, the family and themselves which are inflexible and unrealistic. This may inhibit spontaneity and impede the development of a sensitive spiritual relationship.

25. Caregivers and health care institutions should temper spiritual goals with realism.

26. Ongoing involvement with dying and bereaved persons may cause a severe drain of energy and uncover old and new spiritual issues for the caregiver.

26. Ongoing spiritual education growth, and renewal, should be a part of a staff support program, as well as a personal priority for each caregiver.

COMMUNITY COORDINATION

27. Spiritual resources are available within the community and can make a valuable contribution to the care of the dying patient.	27. Spiritual counsellors from the community should be integral members of the caregiving team.
28. No one caregiver can be expected to understand or address all the spiritual concerns of patients and families.	28. Staff members addressing the needs of patients and families should utilize spiritual resources and caregivers available in the community.

EDUCATION AND RESEARCH

29. Contemporary education for health care professionals often lacks reference to the spiritual dimension of care.	29. Health care curricula should foster an awareness of the spiritual dimension in the clinical setting.
30. Education in spiritual care is impeded by a lack of fundamental research.	30. Research about spiritual care is needed to create a foundation of knowledge which will enhance education and enrich and increase the spiritual aspect of the provision of health care.
31. Freedom from bias is a problem in the conduct of research into spiritual care.	31. Research should be carried out into the development and application of valid and reliable measures of evaluation.

International Work Group on Death, Dying and Bereavement: A Statement of Assumptions and Principles Concerning Education About Death, Dying and Bereavement Developed by the Education Work Group of the IWGDDB

Introduction:

Death, dying and bereavement are fundamental and pervasive aspects of the human experience. Individuals and societies can only achieve fullness of living by understanding and appreciating these realities The absence of such understanding and appreciation may result in unnecessary suffering, loss of dignity, alienation, and diminished quality of living.

Therefore, education about death, dying and bereavement is an essential component of the educational process at all levels, both formal and informal.

General Assumptions:

Education about death, dying and bereavement is important for:

1. Optimizing the potential for human development throughout the life span.
2. Understanding the impact of technology on human life.
3. Achieving equitable allocation of scarce socioeconomic resources.
4. Coping with social systems and social changes.
5. Coping with cross-cultural movement and interaction.
6. Helping to cope with global issues, e.g. nuclear processes and dangers, terrorism, war, world hunger, and population growth.

Therefore, education about death, dying and bereavement needs to be directed to all segments of populations worldwide.

Goals:

The aim of education about death, dying and bereavement is to contribute to general education as a basis for personal development and responsible social participation. It must also contribute to the specific education of those who, as a result of personal or professional circumstances, are closely associated with dying, death and bereavement.

The following assumptions and principles have been prepared as an aid for those who are considering planning, or implementing educational programs about death, dying and bereavement. They are intended for those involved in education about death, dying and bereavement in society at large, including local communities and educational systems.

ASSUMPTIONS	PRINCIPLES
1. In the human cycle, encounters with personal mortality, life-threatening situations, dying, loss and bereavement are centrally important.	1. Because of their central importance, addressing such encounters should be integral to education in society at large, local communities and educational systems. Such education should address:

(a) the universality of death (all living things will one day die),
(b) the irreversibility of death (the physical reality of death is permanent), and
(c) the human limitation and vulnerability revealed within such encounters.

2. Encounters with personal morality, life-threatening situations, dying, loss, and bereavement have potentially profound psychological, physical, spiritual, intellectual, behav-ioral, social and cultural impacts upon the individual.

2. Education should address:
(a) the subjective significance of these encounters,
(b) the variety of impacts upon individuals, and
(c) factors influencing the form, strength and duration of these impacts.

3. Death loss and threat to life are often experienced as unpredictable, unchosen and uncontrollable. Still, some forms of choice and control are often possible as persons and societies define appropriate and meaningful responses.

3. Education should:
(a) speak to experiences of helplessness and hopelessness,
(b) identify forces influencing these experiences, and
(c) speak to possible means to counteract such forces, identify possible choices and recover hope through promotion of choice and control where they are possible.

4. The manner of coping with personal mortality, life-threatening situations, dying, loss and bereavement is pivotally important for sustained individual well being and meaningful living.

4. Education should address:
(a) the importance of individual coping,
(b) a range of alternative coping responses,
(c) the fact that for individuals some responses are more effective than others, and
(d) the value of a social support system for effective coping.

5. Awareness of, and sensitivity to, the needs of others who are encountering personal mortality, life-threatening situations, dying, loss and bereavement are fundamental to enhance sustained quality of social life.

5. Education should:
(a) promote awareness and sensitivity to the needs of others encountering death-related phenomena, and
(b) develop abilities to respond effectively in a word and deed to those needs.

6. Because no loss occurs in isolation from these influences, education should:
(a) address the variety of social and cultural influences upon individual and collective responses to death related phenomena,
(b) promote understanding of influences upon the patterns of death and dying themselves within societies, and
(c) promote understanding of global issues (e.g. nuclear processes and dangers, terrorism, war, world hunger, and population growth), their death-related consequences, and alternative approaches.

6. Social context, technology, cultural values, traditions, rituals and policy influence patterns of individual and collective responses to death-related phenomena.

7. People make choices, the consequences of which affect both quality and quantity of life for themselves and for others.

7. Education should:
(a) address moral responsibility for decisions about life and death and related ethical issues, such as,
 (i) accepting or refusing, providing or withholding life-saving treatments,
 (ii) suicide, and
 (iii) active euthanasia.
(b) the rationality of such decisions,
(c) the ethics of such decisions,
(d) the implications of proxy decision making, and
(e) the appropriateness of governmental and institutional policies and practices related to such decision making.

8. A curriculum is a statement of priorities in education.

8. Education should:
(a) draw upon the assumptions and principles contained in this document in setting its priorities,
(b) be based on the current state of knowledge from a variety of disciplines,
(c) integrate theory and practice, and
(d) incorporate emotional support and foster confidence.

9. Individuals bring to their educational programs experiences that have emerged from a diversity of social, cultural and religious backgrounds.	9. Educational approaches should be appropriate to audience, subject matter, context and goals. Education should provide for: (a) appreciation and utilization of individual differences, (b) sharing of experiences, and (c) promotion of personal growth.
10. Individuals have a range of exposure and responses to loss and death-related experiences.	10. Education needs to develop appropriate strategies to increase exposure to loss and death- related experiences. Educators have a responsibility to anticipate and be sensitive to the death-related experiences of their students, and be prepared to provide appropriate support.
11. Encounters with loss and other death-related phenomena are a part of human experience from earliest childhood.	11. Education for dealing with death-related experiences should begin in early childhood and become an integral part of formal education.
12. Individual's understanding and patterns of coping with loss-related experiences vary along the life span.	12. Whatever the context, education should: (a) reflect sensitivity to level of intellectual development, and (b) support the development of coping capacities in an age-appropriate manner.
13. Individuals who offer informal and formal education in this field provide instruction to teach children and adults about encounters with personal mortality, life-threatening situations, dying, loss and bereavement.	13. Preparation for these responsibilities in informal and formal education about death, dying and bereavement should: (a) promote awareness of, and sensitivity to, the distinctive needs and responsibilities of the diverse populations served, (b) develop knowledge bases appropriate to distinctive instructional missions, and (c) develop skills essential to effective instruction.

14. Research and evaluation are means for assessing the effectiveness of educational efforts.

14. Research should systematically describe the educational process in the field of death, dying and bereavement to permit replication of successful educational efforts. Research should examine the effect of education about death, dying and bereavement on knowledge, attitudes and behaviours. Research findings should be used to revise educational efforts in order to improve their effectiveness.

A Statement of Assumptions and Principles

Concerning Education about Death, Dying and Bereavement for Professionals in Health Care and Human Services.

Developed by the Education Work Group of the Interactional Work Group on Death, Dying and Bereavement

Introduction

These assumptions and principles are intended as an aid for those concerned with education about death, dying and bereavement for professionals in health care and human services.

This education is designed for a wide range of occupations and roles. These include both those who have direct responsibility for the care of individuals and families coping with life- threatening situations, dying and bereavement, as well as those who have indirect or occasional responsibility in such circumstances.

ASSUMPTIONS	PRINCIPLES
1. Services and resources allocated to those who are coping with life-threatening situations, dying and bereavement reflect basic values of individuals, society and the health care system.	1. Education about dying, death and bereavement should be a required, distinct and substantive part of the core education of all health care and human service professionals.
2. A curriculum is a statement of priorities in education.	

3. Health care and human service professionals have a variety of fundamental and inescapable roles to play in the care of individuals and families coping with life-threatening situations, dying and bereavement.	3. Education about death, dying and bereavement should: (a) be based on the current state of knowledge from a variety of disciplines, (b) integrate theory and practice, (c) promote sensitivity, awareness and skills development through role modelling and supervised practise, and (d) provide emotional support and foster confidence.
4. The public has a right to expect that health care and human service professionals will be able to respond effectively in caring for the dying and the bereaved.	
5. Individuals bring to their educational programs experiences that have emerged from a diversity of social, cultural and religious backgrounds.	5. Education about death, dying and bereavement should provide for: (a) appreciation and utilization of individual differences, (b) sharing of experiences, and (c) promotion of personal growth.
6. Individuals will have a range of exposure and responses to loss and death-related experiences.	6. Education about death, dying and bereavement needs to develop appropriate strategies to increase exposure to loss and death-related experiences. Educators have a responsibility to anticipate and be sensitive to the death-related experiences of their students, and be prepared to provide appropriate support.
7. Care of individuals and families who are coping with life-threatening situations, dying and bereavement requires the involvement and cooperation of personnel from many disciplines.	7. Education about death, dying and bereavement should be interdisciplinary in nature, that is, it should examine perspectives from different disciplines and demonstrate relationships among

8. Health care and human service professionals have a long-term impact on the care of individuals and families who are coping with life-threatening situations, dying and bereavement through their involvement in health care and human service systems, and by their roles in educating the next generation of health care and human service professionals.

8. Education about death, dying and bereavement should:
(a) include awareness of how social context, values and policy making influence such care, and
(b) foster the ability of health care and human service professionals to serve as agents for constructive change.

9. The ability to help others also involves the ability to help oneself.

9. Education about death, dying and bereavement should:
(a) enhance the ability of professionals to identify and meet their own needs, and
(b) provide an awareness of the resource available to professionals for their own use.

10. Changes in society and in the context for health care and human services are never- ending, even as exploration of issues related to death, dying and bereavement is ongoing.

10. Continuing education about death, dying and bereavement is necessary to respond to social changes and to address developments in death-related issues.

11. Individuals who offer formal or clinical education in the field of death, dying and bereavement provide instruction to prepare health care and human service professionals for their death-related roles.

11. Preparation for individuals who assume responsibilities for offering formal or clinical education in the field of death, dying and bereavement should:
(a) promote awareness of, and sensitivity to, distinctive needs and responsibilities of the diverse populations to be served,
(b) develop knowledge bases appropriate to distinctive instructional missions, and
(c) develop skills essential to effective instruction.

12. Research is required to evaluate varying strategies for education about death, dying and bereavement for health care and human service professionals.

12. Research should systematically describe the process of education about death, dying and bereavement in order to permit replication of successful programs.

13. Research is required to evaluate the effectiveness of education about death, dying and bereavement in meeting its goals.

13. Research findings should be used to revise educational programs about death, dying and bereavement in order to improve their effectiveness and outcomes. Research should examine effects of education about death, dying and bereavement on outcomes for the dying and the bereaved. Research should examine the effects of education about death, dying and bereavement on knowledge, attitudes and behaviours of health care and human service providers.

Index

Eulogies

Selected passages from tributes to Dr. Dorothy C. H. Ley at her funeral in Beaverton and, later, at her memorial service at St. James Cathedral in Toronto.

The Right Reverend Geoffrey Parke-Taylor, M.A., D.D.
Suffragan Bishop of Toronto (retired)

This is a very sad time for all of us, especially for Dr. Dorothy Ley's family and a wide circle of friends. Many have travelled long distances to be present at this service today. Faithful vigil at her bedside was kept by Norma and Bill, Marlene and Steve, Barbara, Peter, Susie, Betty, Charlotte, Dorothy, Anne, Doreen and many others – as well as the care given by doctors, nurses and clergy. She received visits from our Area Bishop, Bishop Blackwell; Bishop Finlay, our Diocesan Bishop, drove up from Toronto as recently as Saturday [a few days before her death] to see her, bless her, and bid her farewell. This has been a wonderful demonstration of what it means to care – palliative care at its best, fully in accord with what Dorothy herself taught and practised.

This is indeed a time of sadness for members of this parish and this community. Yet this is also a time for profound and joyful thanksgiving. We give thanks for Dorothy's life and distinguished career as a physician, active member of the church and leader in the community.

The two words which best describe Dorothy's long struggle with cancer are courage and faith. She has faced surgery, radiation and chemotherapy with great courage, continuing with all her many commitments and responsibilities well beyond the call of duty, relinquishing them only when she no longer had the physical strength to carry on. Her faith has always been her main resource, a deep and abiding faith which sustained her and give her special courage. She knew full well that God has made us not for this life only but for all eternity. For her, life was to be lived under the sovereignty of Jesus Christ, who is Lord of all. His victory over death is now the supreme reality, as she lives for evermore in His presence.

Bishop Brent, born in Canada, and a leader in the ecumenical movement, has this to say about life beyond death: "What is dying? I am standing on a shore. A ship sails to the morning breeze and starts for the ocean. She is an object of beauty and I stand watching her till at last she fades on the horizon and someone at my side says, 'She is gone' – Gone where? Gone from my sight, that is all. She is just as she was when I saw her, and just as able to bear her load of living freight to its destination. The diminished size and total loss of sight is in me, not in her; and just at the moment when someone at my side says, 'She is gone' – there are others who are watching her coming, and other voices on another shore take up a glad shout, 'Here she comes' – and that, that is dying."

We rejoice as we entrust Dorothy into the infinite care of God and the peace and love which know no ending.

Dr. Larry Librach
Director, Division of Palliative Medicine
Mount Sinai Hospital, Toronto

In my Jewish faith, there is a tradition in our teachings saying that each person has three names:

1. The name we are born with, i.e. the name of our ancestors – it signifies our heritage,
2. The name our parents give us, i.e. the part of our personhood that derives from what our parents teach us and how we are moulded by our family,
3. Finally, the name we make for ourselves as we travel the journey of life.

My role today is to briefly describe the name that Dr. Dorothy Ley made for herself in the area of palliative care.

Dorothy used to delight in telling people that she taught me everything that I know. I was a student of hers in my third year of undergraduate medicine. I then was privileged to work with her when I was an intern at Toronto Western Hospital. I remember her well. She was a thorough and very knowledgeable physician who was dedicated to her patients. She always expressed considerable concern for the terminally-ill cancer patients she served as a haematologist-oncologist. These were the days that so many terminally-ill cancer patients were treated almost as pariahs in hospitals. Dorothy at that time was known for her devotion and humanity towards these patients and she expected the same from interns and residents who trained with her.

The important projects that she began and completed during her tenure as president of the [Palliative Care] Foundation included:

- the *Palliative Care Directory*
- the palliative care resource centre; a centralized collection of educational materials of all sorts intended as a national resource
- the founding of the biennial National Palliative Care Conferences
- the founding of the *Journal of Palliative Care*
- a series of Pain Control seminars across Canada
- multiple public forums to disseminate information about palliative care all across Canada
- planning consultations for the establishment of palliative care services and programs across Canada
- many different speaking engagements on the topic of palliative care
- advocacy at government and at organizational levels
- building bridges internationally in the field of palliative care.

Dorothy experienced first hand the need for adequate Home Care services when she looked after [her cousin] Donnie at home. She then became even more committed to developing home-based palliative care services. She directed the task force on palliative care for the Metro Toronto District Health Council through its 18 months of deliberations even though she was weakened by her disease and often in considerable distress from her disease and the chemotherapy.

One of the legacies of Dorothy's involvement in palliative care is, of course, the hospice that bears her name. I remember her calling me once about some matter and at the end of the call asking me my advice about the proposal to name a hospice program after her. She wondered whether she had made that much of contribution to deserve such an honour. Frankly, the other thing that bothered her was the fact as she expressed it, that, "I'm not dead yet! Why do they want to do this anyway?" However, she allowed the hospice to be named after her and it will survive as one of the memorials to her.

These few words are a brief testimony to our colleague and friend, Dr. Dorothy Ley, and her involvement in palliative care. I will remember her for her warmth. I will remember her for the courage she showed during her cancer illness. I will remember her for her dogged determination and dedication to the development of palliative care.

We will all remember her for her contributions as one of the founders and pioneers of palliative care in Canada. May she rest well and in peace in the hands of G-d.

Elizabeth Latimer, M.D., C.C.F.P., F.C.F.P.
Representing the Ontario Medical Association

It is an honour to remember Dr. Dorothy Ley whom I knew as a colleague, friend, role model and mentor. As a colleague, Dorothy was a physician in the true sense of the word. She cared about people – her patients and her colleagues. Throughout her career, she made herself available to patients for the alleviation of their suffering.

Dorothy always worked towards excellence and espoused and, indeed lived, the values of integrity and true dignity. She truly believed in whole-person care – caring for the person, not the "patient" or the "disease". In her work, she truly believed in interdisciplinary care, valuing the involvement of every profession and person who could help.

Dorothy spoke accurately and eloquently in support of effective care of the dying in Canada. She continually challenged large organizations and health care systems to assume their rightful role and responsibility for this care. She spoke openly and honestly for the values and standards of care in which she believed.

For me personally, Dorothy represented an exemplary role model of a female physician; someone who practised with energy, skill and dedication; someone who was able to achieve admirable levels of effectiveness, locally, nationally and internationally and never lost her sense of herself. Truly she was a pioneer in Canada, as a woman and as a physician.

As a friend, I always admired Dorothy's courage, her candour, her faith and her sense of humour and fun. I know that these qualities, combined with her love of her home, family and friends and her little dog, helped to carry her through her illness. Dorothy possessed a remarkable sensitivity to the poignancy and power of our shared human situation. We will miss her.

Reverend Douglas Graydon
Coordinator, Counselling Services
Casey House Hospice, Toronto

How is one supposed to feel when a mentor dies? I have known Dorothy for may years. She and I share Christian roots and she had a powerful presence within the Anglican Church.

I first heard of Dorothy at a workshop on palliative care: I can't remember where or when, but I do remember her encouraging my interest in palliative care, its philosophy and development. I remember her passion and dedication towards maintaining the integrity, dignity and autonomy of patients. I remember her gentleness and sensitivity. And I also remember her impatience with her own profession as she struggled to teach other physicians the importance of tending not only to the physical pain of their patients, but the emotional and spiritual pain as well.

Dorothy was active in the creation of Casey House Hospice; the only free-standing AIDS hospice in Canada. She was one of our first members of the Board of Directors and contributed to shaping Casey House into what it is today.

Dorothy and I, however, worked most closely together on the Anglican Church's AIDS Committee. She struggled with the Diocese of Toronto as it tried to articulate its pastoral response to

AIDS. She was an extraordinary resource and was one of the principal architects in formulating a church response which will grow and develop into the future because of her contribution.

Dorothy's dedication to better society was felt in many ways. One such example was her quiet commitment to the growth and development of THE TERESA GROUP, the only community-based volunteer organization in Canada which provides emotional and practical support to families with HIV positive children.

Dorothy Ley was a mentor of mine. She embodied a sense of compassion and commitment which I admired. She pushed me into areas and realms of challenge and learning which have taught me lessons which will stand the test of time. She changed my perceptions and deepened my understanding of palliative care, faith and what it means to serve humanity.

I will miss Dorothy's knowledge, her humour, her gentle ways. I will miss sitting in her yard on the shores of Lake Simcoe discussing medicine, theology and "life in general". I will, however, always celebrate the fact that she was part of my life.

Homily given by the **Right Reverend Terence E. Finlay**
Bishop of Toronto

Dorothy Ley touched all of us in a variety of ways. This afternoon we have heard some of these wonderful stories. For me she possessed an intuitive sense of when to be present, when to call, when to care for another. I am sure that each of you could add many more stories. For many of us, within the context of the Christian community, she was a woman of faith, of conviction, a follower of Jesus Christ. Last Wednesday, Ash Wednesday, we participated in a strange tradition, for some, of having the sign of the cross made on our foreheads in the ashes which come from the burning of the Palm branches from Palm Sunday last year. It reminded us of our mortality, "out of dust were we created and to dust we shall return," but also it recalled our baptism when we are signed with the cross and marked as Christ's own forever. The cross is a sign of our identity. A mark of those who identify, whose life and work are tied to the person and work of Jesus Christ:

- a life proclaiming good news
- a life of living reconciliation
- a life of welcoming, befriending, of reaching out and loving others.

Yes, a life that leads to death, but beyond death, to resurrection.

Dorothy's life proclaimed good news. She worked to bring healing and life. She lived by reaching out in concern and compassion for others. In a death-denying, death-avoiding society, Dorothy has much to teach us.

Those who were with her during those last hours know that it was with a quiet confidence and radiant serenity that she boldly faced up to that which the world spends so much time and money running away from. I am sure it was not easy for her to face her own death, because she spent so much of her life working to preserve the lives of others. But she was able to do so, not so much because she believed in eternal life, but because she had a bold, confident faith in the eternal love of God. Dorothy's hope as she faced death was the same hope which sustains the Christian throughout life; that the God who has created us and claimed us from our birth, the God who loves us and grasps us in life, will continue to claim us and love us and grasp us, even in death.

And so we commend to the care of a loving and faithful creator, the soul of our friend Dorothy Ley, a cherished child of God, who bore on her brow and in her life the sign of the cross – marked as Christ's own forever.

Rest eternal grant unto her, O Lord and let light perpetual shine upon her. May she rest in peace. Amen.

The following Psalm 23 was read at Dr. Ley's funeral held at St. Paul's Anglican Church in Beaverton, Ontario on February 3, 1994.

The Lord is my shepherd;
I shall not want.
He maketh me to lie down in green pastures;
He leadeth me beside the still waters.
He restoreth my soul;
He leadeth me in the paths
of righteousness for his name's sake.
Yea, though I walk
through the valley of the shadow of death,
I will fear no evil;
for Thou are with me;
Thy rod and Thy staff they comfort me.
Thou preparest a table before me
in the presence of mine enemies;
Thou annointest my head with oil;
my cup runneth over.
Surely goodness and mercy
shall follow me all the days of my life:
and I will dwell in the
house of the Lord for ever.